ERG-ONOMIC LIVING

HOW TO CREATE A USER-FRIENDLY HOME AND OFFICE

GORDON INKELES AND IRIS SCHENCKE

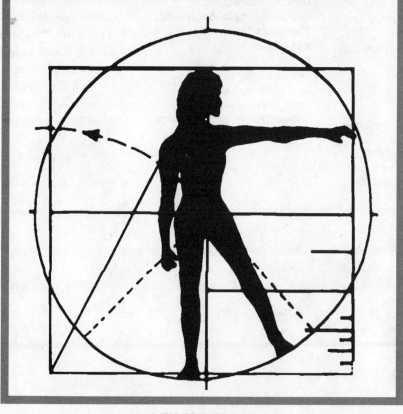

A FIRESIDE BOOK
PUBLISHED BY SIMON & SCHUSTER
New York | London | Toronto | Sydney | Tokyo | Singapore

FIRESIDE
Rockefeller Center
1230 Avenue of the Americas
New York, New York 10020

The Richard Brautigan poem
"All Watched Over by Machines of
Loving Grace" from *The Pill Versus
the Springhill Mining Disaster*,
Dell Publishing Company, Inc.,
New York, 1968, has been reprinted
by permission of the author's estate.

Designed by Jon Goodchild
at NVision³.
Illustrated by Karla Kaizoji Austin,
John Rutherford and Laura Zerzan.

Manufactured in the United States
of America

10 9 8 7 6 5 4 3 2 1

LIBRARY OF CONGRESS
CATALOGING-IN-PUBLICATION DATA
Inkeles, Gordon.
    Ergonomic living: how to
create a user-friendly home and
office/Gordon Inkeles and Iris
Schencke.
    P.   cm.
    1. House furnishings.
    2. Human engineering.
    3. Office furniture.
    I. Schencke, Iris.
    II. Title.
TX311.I58   1994
    645 — dc20
                94 – 7888

ISBN 0-02-093081-X

The authors are grateful for
permission to use photos from
the following manufacturers of
ergonomic products:

AliMed® Inc.
Anthro Corporation
Apple Computer, Inc.
Armstrong World Industries, Inc.
Bang & Olufsen
Brookstone
Canon USA, Inc.
Compaq Computer Corporation
Duxiana/Dux Interiors, Inc.
Ekornes
Herman Miller Corporation
Hewlett Packard
IBM Corporation
IKEA
Interior Acoustics, Inc.
Kensington
Keytime
The Knoll Group
Koss Corporation
Levenger Company
Luxo Corporation
North Coast Medical, Inc.
Olympus America Inc.
Optical Coating Laboratory, Inc.
Plantronics, Inc.
Radio Shack
Radius Inc.
Self Care Catalog
Sony Electronics Inc.
Tandy Corporation
Texwood Furniture Corporation
Unifor, Francesco Radino

Special thanks from Iris Schencke
to:
    Alan Purchase, a fine communi-
cator who showed me that even the
lowly typewriter can be interesting.
    Jacques Vallee, who lived well
in the information habitat when it
was in its infancy.
    Steve Jobs, who, in typical
fashion, went from skeptic to
advocate and in a few months
introduced ergonomic design at
Apple Computer.
    Both authors are grateful to
Karla Kaizoji Austin, John
Rutherford and Laura Zerzan for
their excellent illustrations and to
Emily Guthrie and Mel Lockey for
their insights on childhood
ergonomics. We would also like
to thank Mark Chimsky, who
believed in this book from the
outset, Jon Goodchild for his book
organization and design, Scott
Harrison and our incomparable
agent, Elaine Markson.

*This book is not intended as a
substitute for the medical advice
of physicians. The reader should
regularly consult a physician in
matters relating to his or her health
and particularly with regard to
any symptoms that may require
diagnosis or medical attention.*

To my mother,
Kerstin Lindqvist,
with love.
—IRIS SCHENCKE

To Lee Wakefield,
for his vision
and enduring
friendship.
—GORDON INKELES

All Watched Over by Machines of Loving Grace

I like to think (and
the sooner the better!)
of a cybernetic meadow
where mammals and computers
live together in mutually
programming harmony
like pure water
touching clear sky.

I like to think
   (right now, please!)
of a cybernetic forest
filled with pines and electronics
where deer stroll peacefully
past computers
as if they were flowers
with spinning blossoms.

I like to think
   (it has to be!)
of a cybernetic ecology
where we are free of our labors
and joined back to nature,
returned to our mammal
brothers and sisters,
and all watched over
by machines of loving grace.

— RICHARD BRAUTIGAN

Contents

Habitat: Your Personal Space

here is a kind of habitat of man-made objects around you, where you live and work. It can be hostile or friendly. It determines whether you are exhausted and cranky at the end of the day or still fairly fresh. It works with you or against you. It can be healthful or it can batter you with headaches, eyestrain, backaches and other pain. ❦ What makes the difference, what makes a user-friendly human habitat, is good ergonomics. ❦ Ergonomics is the relationship of furniture and tools to your own body. A chair that fits your body allows you to sit for hours in comfort. That seems simple enough—until you try to buy one. Unfortunately, most furniture is designed to match other furniture and not your body. ❦ Simply making do with things as they are carries a price. Do you find work stressful? Do you have trouble unwinding when you get home? Are you suffering from nonspecific aches and pains, bizarre allergies? Don't blame yourself; the problem could be in the places where you spend your time. ❦ If you work in an overlighted office filled with noisy machinery and sleep on a superhard mattress, you're already making too many compromises. And if you're struggling to relax in amorphous sofas, wedging yourself into chairs and cubicles that seem to be getting more cramped and less comfortable every time you sit down, your body is under constant stress. Your habitat, whether at home or at work, isn't yours. ❦ Ergonomics shows you how to reclaim it, using your own body as the true measure of your needs. This is a health book, but there are no tedious exercises to learn, no time-consuming meditations, no impossible diets, no sacrifices. To make informed ergonomic choices about your home and office habitats, you need only permit yourself to *feel* what's right. ❦ Since every action has a price that must be paid by your muscles and nerves, the ergonomic choice is always the healthiest one. In time, the wrong chair, desk, lighting or bed will undo the beneficial effects of daily exercise and undermine the healthiest lifestyle. You can adjust to uncomfortable working conditions for an hour or two, but if a task must be repeated regularly, the ergonomic factor makes the difference between a dull, aching body and an alert, rested one. Ergonomics provides the missing link in the modern health equation: control over the external environment where health problems originate.

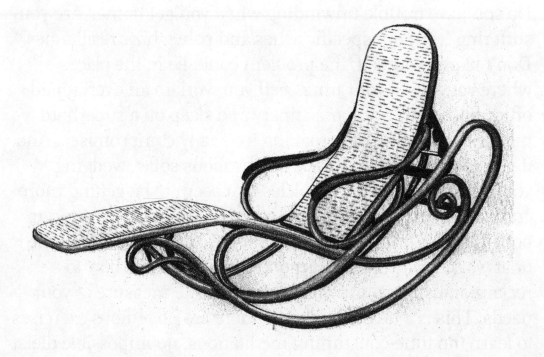

Ergonomic Resources

You don't need a battery of laboratory tests in order to select a bed or desk; the message you get from your own body matters more. The whole point of this book is that you can decide for yourself which items fit your body properly. Once you understand that whether you're preparing a meal, operating a computer or watching television, you have a right to clean air, decent lighting and proper lumbar support, you'll begin to see products differently. A few manufacturers have had their priorities right from the beginning, emphasizing ergonomics instead of the sheer number of features. You can feel the difference.

Throughout the book, we've included various ergonomics resources. Our recommendations are meant as starting points from which you can make your own choices. However, should you decide to use the book as a shopping guide, you won't be disappointed. The ergonomic choice is almost always better made and more pleasing than the competition. Sharp edges, whining fans and intimidating remotes give way to buttons and handles that fit your hand, machines that run silently and controls that are well-marked and logical. What all these products have in common is the idea that good design starts with an understanding of human physiology, and just as bodies differ, the things we use must be flexible as well. The benefit to the user is immediately apparent: an easy motion is a healthful one; an awkward motion can make you sore in minutes.

Flipping through these pages, you will discover a new way of looking at the world, one that dispenses with hype and advertising claims once and for all. You will also encounter the ergonomic aesthetic: a look of quality and human-centered engineering.

But we urge you to take it a step further. Go out and *try* the ergonomic alternative. Feel the difference, then make your choice

 Ergonomic resource icon

How to Use This Book

Use the ergonomic programs here to identify hidden sources of stress at home and at work. Get rid of the *things* that cause stress in your life.

Initially, ergonomic advantages may appear insignificant; after all, most kitchens are functional, the most primitive computer is faster than your old typewriter, and almost any bed will do when you are exhausted. But one day means nothing if you spend thousands of hours a year being uncomfortable. As the effects of glare, noise and pressure accumulate, your body will pay the inevitable price.

If you've already started paying, ergonomic choices are an antidote to panic. Do you have trouble focusing your eyes at the end of the day? Are you plagued by headaches and lower-back pain that seem to get worse the moment you sit down? Are you constantly interrupted at work? Perhaps you have a specific health concern: you might be pregnant and concerned about radiation from your computer screen. Working with the computer seems to require some kind of filter—but which one? Are you looking for a more restful bed, a truly comfortable reading chair, a more efficient kitchen layout?

Think of the familiar and necessary items in your daily life: mattress, kitchen sink, office chair and so on. Then consider for a moment just how much time you spend with each of these things every day. Finally, make a list of your health problems that don't seem to be related to any illness or injury. With this rough inventory of priorities and problems in hand, look up the items in this book that determine the comfort of your daily existence. A general discussion of design and health problems followed by straightforward, ergonomic solutions accompanies each item.

Use this book as a shopping guide to select ergonomic products for your personal habitats. Forget the tedious sales brochures and the charts of technical specifications. You'll learn where a chair is actually supposed to support your back, which controls you really need to see when operating an entertainment system (and which are distracting) and how to select a mattress that enhances your personal sleep patterns. If you sleep better, you'll be more productive at work, and your backache will disappear.

Use this book as a tool to transform your life, to turn a hostile place into a friendly habitat. You don't need a lot of money or special approval from the boss to make most ergonomic changes.

You need information.

HOME

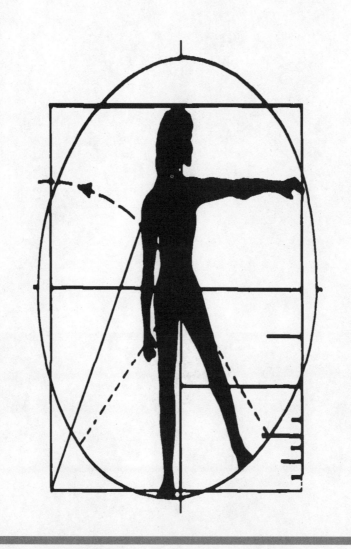

The Ergonomic Home

Your home is your most personal habitat, a space to relax, play and work in peace. You've got to be able to find peace of mind here at the end of the day—not waste time kicking your way through clutter in a hostile place that fights you every step of the way. Your body suffers enough insults daily; you cannot afford to make compromises in your own kitchen and bedroom. You deserve an accommodating home, a friendly place where everything works almost intuitively. ❧ Making your home or apartment ergonomic is a simple process with instant rewards—you will see changes in people the first day. You don't need an interior decorator or a house full of sleek, minimalist gadgetry to make it happen. Traditional furniture like rocking chairs and four-legged step stools work as well as, and sometimes better than, ultramodern "designer" items. And you don't have to rip apart your home to make it ergonomic. Sometimes merely rearranging the furniture will revolutionize the way your family eats, talks and plays together. The changes aren't costly, although as you become more attuned to the ergonomic life you may wish to replace a few items of furniture that you never liked and never knew why. ❧ Ergonomics takes the stress out of shopping for your home. You begin to look at products differently, dispensing once and for all with bewildering manufacturers' hype. You learn to ask the crucial ergonomic questions: Will I understand intuitively how an item works? Will a stranger know what it's for? Will it make life easier and more comfortable? When you touch an ergonomic product, you should be able to see and feel the difference. ❦ An ergonomic home changes the way people behave—starting with yourself. When you sit down to read or watch television you will have no urge to rearrange the furniture. You will sleep better every night on an ergonomic bed, and you will feel the difference the next day. Others benefit too. In the child-friendly home, children begin to eat quietly with the family, help out in the kitchen and read independently. Chores that once caused arguments become more democratic. Housework turns into an obvious process that is everybody's responsibility rather than the domain of a single, frazzled family member. Work becomes less specialized and more enjoyable. A friend can drop by, walk right into the kitchen and begin cooking without a frantic search through every drawer and cupboard. Everything works. ❦ As ergonomic solutions spread through your home, unprecedented social exchanges begin to occur. Arguments over missing clothes and lost items no longer erupt. Leisure time leaves you feeling rested and energetic. Conversation replaces compulsive television watching, parties become relaxed and enjoyable. Guests who once clustered at the dining room table suddenly wander into the living room, smiling. Your home acquires a friendly ambience that makes everyone feel welcome. It's a warm, inviting place, a human-centered sanctuary. ❦ But you live there; you know.

1. How to Enter Your Home

The traditional home entrance with coat closet, hall table and mirror comes to us courtesy of the nineteenth century, when life was much less complicated. In those days people had one or two pairs of shoes, a hat for each season and a sturdy umbrella. They received a couple of letters a day and tossed all their garbage into a pail under the sink. ❧ Things came and went in the home under the watchful eye of a housewife or housekeeper who was always on hand to gather up the loose odds and ends. She made the home *seem* ergonomic even if it wasn't. ❧ A hundred years later we have managed to complicate with an astonishing array of possessions what was once a predictable environment. The hall closet is usually full a day after we move in, and the housewife hurries off to the office the next morning. The hall table cannot accommodate today's gigantic set of phone books, much less the stylish telephone and answering machine. We consider eliminating the table altogether and simply hanging the phone on the wall. ❧ Then we turn our attention from the entrance to the rest of the home.

Entry Ergonomics

Entry mats

Storage for shoes, coats, hats, umbrellas

Sports rack

Cubbies

Sorting table

Mail tower

Recycling

The Storm at Your Front Door

We set up furniture, appliances, carpets and lighting. We painstakingly match chairs and tables and then we add dashes of color—plants and art—until each room looks appealing.

Meanwhile, back at the front door, an insidious process has begun that will undermine all our attempts to create a pleasant environment. Mountains of coats, shoes, toys, sports equipment, office work, groceries, packing materials, mail, junk mail and rubble surge past the overflowing hall closet into our carefully decorated home. No room is spared, and no shelf, ledge, couch, bed, chair back, table, carpet, door back or desk is exempted. If we are in denial about the mess itself, we argue constantly about the stressful side effects of living in chaos. The unruly state of our possessions has become a major domestic crisis. Marriages flounder over much less dramatic issues than sex, money and power; they collapse slowly under the demoralizing effects of bad ergonomics.

Women resent the second shift they are expected to work in the home. Men, of course, resent it just as much if they end up organizing endless piles of other people's stuff. We cannot know how many marriage counselors have wrestled vainly with housework plans, steadfastly rearranging the deck chairs amid an accelerating storm of litter, while the marriage ungracefully sinks. But the crisis is ergonomic, not psychological: our homes are no longer set up to manage our possessions. So many "small things" that seem to start the most terrible arguments—persistent piles of junk, lost possessions, dripping raincoats in the living room—boil down to ergonomic failures. Yes, each family member must take responsibility for managing his or her own loading and unloading chores. That single change can indeed transform a bickering family into a tranquil one. But we cannot take the first step without decentralizing the management process.

While being at home does not demand acting as an efficiency expert (a cure worse than the problem), you have a lot to gain by spending an hour planning how to manage the flow of objects in and out of your home. Many items scattered around your residence shouldn't have gotten past the entrance.

Most homes have a second entrance for family use, an ideal spot for loading and unloading. Reserve the formal entrance for guests. If you don't have a second entrance, add as many of this section's suggestions as possible just inside your front door. Recommendations for the family entrance—sports racks, shoe racks and so on—also work well in an attached garage, which is the main loading and unloading entrance in many suburban homes.

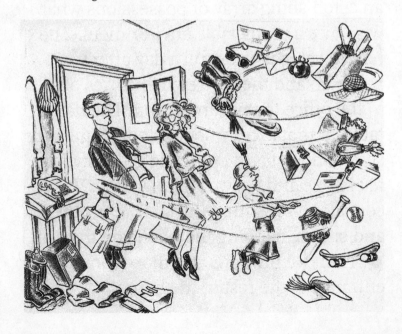

Think of the entrance as a mud room: a barrier between the dirt and clutter from the outside world and your home. It is also a place to sort and store things like umbrellas, gym bags and dog leashes that travel in and out of your home frequently. If the ergonomic entrance accomplishes nothing else, it will eliminate those frantic searches for lost items that always seem to occur minutes before an appointment. Mom was once expected to take responsibility for storing everything that flew through the front door. With an ergonomic storage plan, however, the familiar demand "Where's my homework, lunch, briefcase, pocket book?" vanishes. Each family member finds it easy to be responsible for his or her own things.

This section of the book presents a complete loading and unloading plan for the entry to your home. Fully executed, the plan will make life noticeably easier for everyone in your family. Without such a plan anyone who enters your home ends up doing extra work.

Entry Mats

People expect to wipe their feet before entering your home. Why not make it a meaningful experience? Entry mats are your initial barrier against the outside world. Take the mats seriously because any dirt that gets past them ends up inside your home.

Two mats intercept far more dirt than one. Most shoes have layered dirt deposits that won't come off with a single wiping. Use a corrugated rubber mat outside the door for serious foot scraping and pounding. As mud and thick dirt come off the shoes, it falls through the corrugations. Interior mats must stay in place to be useful. Place your second mat, made from nonslip rubber-backed cloth, just inside the door where it can absorb the light dirt that the thicker mat misses.

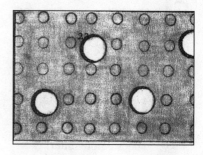

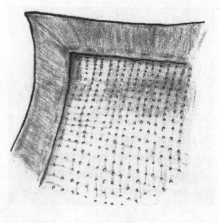

Dirt barriers, outside and inside

Brookstone
1655 Bassford Drive
Mexico, Missouri 65265
(800) 926 7000

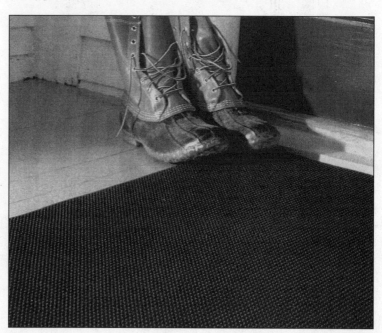

Shoes, Coats, Hats and Umbrellas

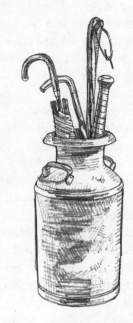

Taking off your outside shoes before entering a home, an eminently civilized Japanese and Swedish custom, preserves an effective dirt barrier at the front door. The ergonomic payoff: your entire home stays noticeably cleaner, and you have less housework to do. Wear slippers indoors whenever possible; you'll love them. Keeping a couple of pairs of indoor and outdoor shoes on a wooden or metal shoe stand just inside the door makes the dirt barrier easy to use. Use a simple, straightforward stand—nothing difficult to balance, no precisely fitted shoe slots. Make it quick and easy to exchange shoes at the front door. Keep a stool on hand to make your guests comfortable during changing. Be generous with your slippers but be reasonable. Not every guest will want to remove his or her shoes at your door. Keep an extra pair of slippers on hand for those who do.

Hang coats and hats that you wear daily in a visible spot. Never stuff them into a closet next to things you wear twice a year. Set up a coat and flat hat rack that accommodates everybody. Children will require a separate coat and hat rack placed within their reach. They will then happily manage their own clothes (just like the grownups!) instead of flinging them onto the floor and expecting you to take over.

Store umbrellas visibly in a separate container, never in the back of a closet. Buy an old-fashioned stand or set aside an upright container (like the milk can pictured here) for umbrellas and walking sticks. This works much better than any hook or hanger and keeps water from spreading on rainy days. Umbrellas must be ready to go when you are.

 Carlson Wood Products
Miranda, California 95553
(707) 943 3398

 Neil C. Elmer
Potter Valley,
California 95469

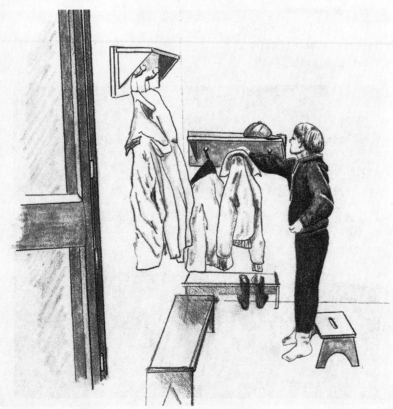

Sports Rack

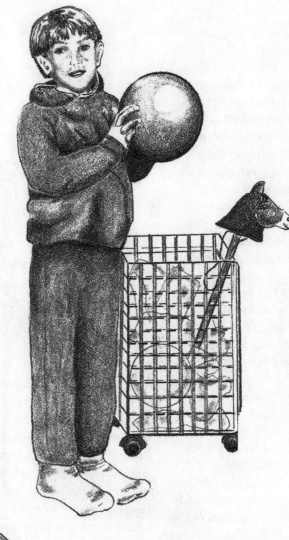

Basketballs in the hall make for challenging late-night trips to the bathroom. A wire sports rack hung just inside the back door or garage gives your children, instead of you, a place to keep their equipment. A large upper rack accommodates footballs, basketballs and soccer balls. A smaller lower rack will store baseballs and tennis balls. Hang related sports equipment like mitts and knee pads from the lower rack. Baseball bats hang neatly from a separate holder that clips onto the top rack. If your wall space is limited, a sports corral works well too.

 Design Ideas
6 Fair Oaks
Springfield, Illinois 62704

 Hold Everything
P.O. Box 7807
San Francisco, California 94120
(800) 421 2264

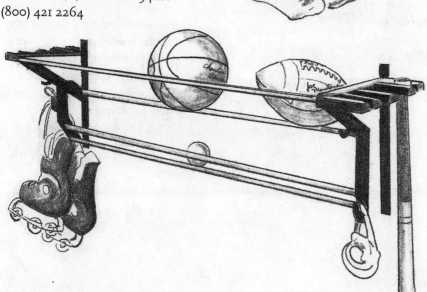

A Cubby for Everyone

Every activity has its bag. Think of the anxiety you will eliminate if every member of your family can find a gym, camera, school or shopping bag when it's needed. Imagine if the lunch box, briefcase, pocketbook or overnight bag stood ready to go next to the door. The cubby is a powerful ergonomic tool that tucks against the wall just inside your door. It will go into use the moment it's finished.

Storing all of your family's bags in a single, large entrance cubby liberates space everywhere in your home. It also saves time and eliminates petty frustrations. Best of all, each individual becomes responsible for storing his or her own possessions. You will never again hear the plaintive "Where did you put my bowling bag?"

Make the cubby out of wooden cubes (see illustration). Be careful not to crowd the cubes—dedicate each one to a different bag. If your family is large, color code the cubes to avoid confusion.

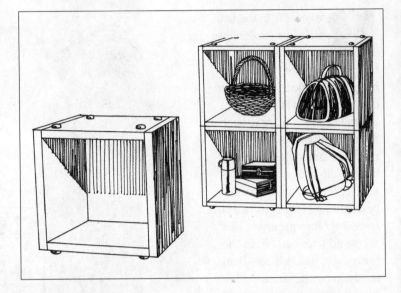

The Sorting Table

When you carry packages or mail into your home, the first thing you want to do is put them down. If you use the kitchen table, you are aiding and abetting the migration of wrapping paper, styrofoam pellets, string ends, plastic tape and used envelopes into your home. Rather than argue about these "insignificant" items with every member of your family, get them out of the way at the entrance to your home.

Set up a sturdy table dedicated to loading and unloading inside your entrance. Since you will put on your hat and comb your hair nearby, hang a mirror above this table. Place a large wastebasket for wrapping material, junk mail and trash under the table. Keep a large scissors nearby.

You will use the sorting table virtually every time you enter your home with bags of groceries, a handful of mail or a package. A week after you set up this fundamental ergonomic tool, you will be wondering where you once *put* things.

Mail Tower

If you live with other people, you need a system to manage mail, lest one individual become responsible for everything (or worse, no one becomes responsible for any of it). We have all seen arguments flare up as neat little stacks of daily mail swell to unmanageable mountains. This is not a failure of organization—you're organized enough at work, you have a right to relax at home. If you allow yourself and your family to be pushed around by the daily mail, ripples of discontent will spread throughout your home. In fact, this is precisely the kind of "insignificant" problem that can spark nasty, recurrent arguments.

If you feel stressed the moment you step into your home, the mail may already be getting the better of you. Instead of focusing on your frustration, look closely at the ergonomics of your entrance. If you're busy, you shouldn't have to sort mail daily, and you shouldn't have to separate your mail from everyone else's. You need a mail tower.

Unfortunately, nobody makes such a product for the home (yet). But you can easily set one up yourself. Shelves must be deep enough for magazines, newspapers and mail. Individual storage systems can vary. You can reserve separate shelves for magazines, newspapers, bills and personal mail or paint color codes on sets of shelves for each individual according to his needs (dad, five blue shelves, daughter, three gold shelves). Occupying little more than a single square foot of floor space, this essential ergonomic tool has a small *footprint*. Five minutes after the mail tower enters your home, your family will start filling it up.

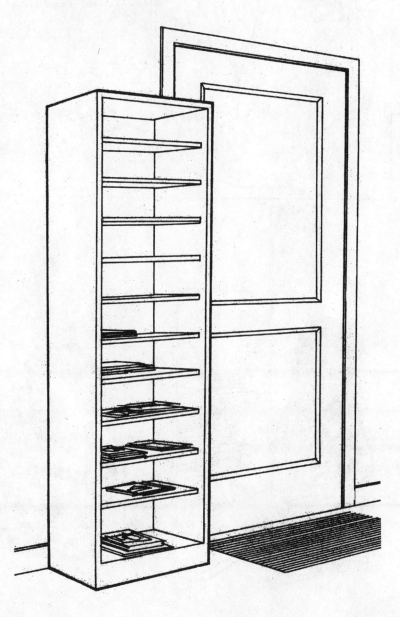

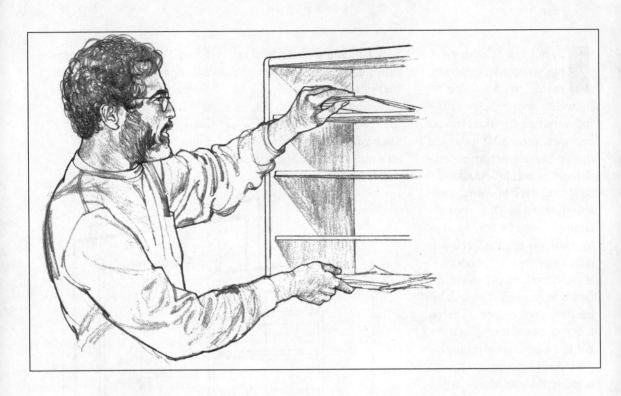

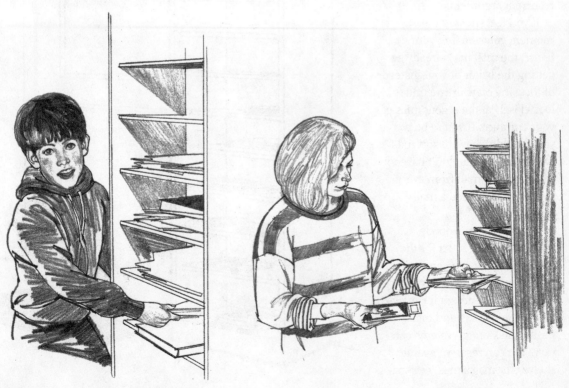

Recycling

Traditional refuse disposal—one bulky, stinking can under the sink—is going the way of the toxic dump: we can't afford it anymore. Bad news for the earth and for us, it didn't require much design, thought or effort. Sloppy garbage handling spoiled us for the work we now have to do.

Recycling has added a half dozen small jobs to home management that simply didn't exist just a few years ago. And each job requires an ergonomic storage plan. Few activities will teach you the value of ergonomics quicker than a haphazard recycling program that simply spreads piles of garbage around the home.

Recycling creates other problems that discourage our best intentions. It takes up considerably more space than the traditional garbage bin and can easily become an eyesore. Beware of the handyman approach to recycling, which

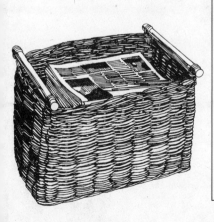

Recycling Shortcuts

Don't reload

Use containers that can go from the collection point to the car, on to the recycling center and then back home again.

Use one hand

Compost buckets and recycling bins should be operated by one hand (or foot). Avoid putting a can or bottle down before placing it in its proper recycling bin.

Stack containers

Be sure you can dispose of a bottle or can without restacking everything. Keep it simple or the containers won't be used.

Keep containers light

Heavy containers will sit in place and overflow.

Easily cleaned

Make sure containers are made of washable material.

Deodorize it

Plain baking soda works better than many commercial cleaners. Avoid complex and costly solutions to simple problems.

Compact and crush

A wall-mounted can crusher and/or a built-in garbage compactor substantially reduce the the volume of your garbage.

Mark containers

Use color coding or pictures to indicate where various wastes belong.

can complicate the process even further. Installing garbage chutes in the walls of your house that feed into basement or backyard compost bins creates a maze of new cleaning responsibilities. Remember: every system you bring into your home requires maintenance. Don't build the system if you aren't ready to maintain it.

Recycling is extra work, but it actually reduces sloppy garbage handling. Sorting out glass, aluminum and paper reduces the load in your main garbage pail. Composting requires a few square feet of yard space. If you haven't got the space, use a garbage disposal unit to get rid of food scraps. Either way, you will end up with garbage that is more sanitary.

 Hold Everything
P.O. Box 7807
San Francisco, California 94120
(800) 421 2264

Note handles on bins

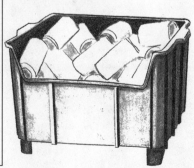

Ergonomic Recycling

Since you must keep each variety of recyclable product in a dedicated container, it's important to eliminate extra steps. Make sure each container is easy to carry—you will need sturdy handles for collections of glass. Keep your recycling containers near the various work areas. If you're remodeling your kitchen, consider built-in containers.

Use containers with built-in casters for heavier items like glass and metal. They can then be rolled out of the way for mopping and out of your home when the time comes.

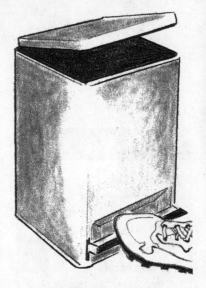

Keep it simple. Before you recycle a single bottle, stop and multiply that bottle by 250. Your recycling program must not include extra steps, or it will soon be abandoned.

The Ergonomic Garbage Pail

A foot-operated lever opens the lid; gravity closes it. An inner plastic container with a handle makes it easy to carry, empty and clean. Set up separate cans for glass, aluminum, plastic and nonrecyclable garbage. Use one foot to operate the can, one hand to carry it.

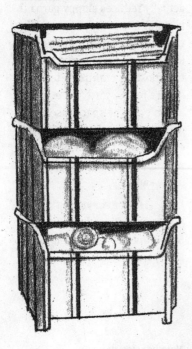

2. The Child-Friendly Home

We've come a long way from the notion that children should be seen and not heard, but we still haven't provided them with the ergonomic tools that adults take for granted. Children's table manners, attention span, handwriting and disposition would improve radically if only their feet were planted firmly on the floor. ❧ Specialized furniture like cribs and high chairs, supplied willingly enough to infants, is abandoned soon after a child begins to walk. At three years of age children are suddenly expected to "adapt" to adult-size furniture. ❧ For years, whole families are caught in the undertow of bad ergonomics, arguing, blaming and apologizing like mad. At the center of the storm, perched on the edge of a giant chair, feet dangling off the floor, is the child who is routinely blamed. We make demands on children that we don't make of ourselves. Try having dinner seated on a drafting stool (skip the footrest), and you will understand how children feel when they are unable to use their feet for balance. ❧ Your child has the same rights to comfort you have and deserves the same ergonomic advantages.

The Independent Child

We all treasure images of a child sitting on the edge of a huge chair, feet dangling far above the ground. We wouldn't smile so readily, however, if we could experience the child's very real ergonomic dilemma. He's stuck in the wrong chair—and we put him there.

We replace a child's clothing because we must. But the child also outgrows elements in his physical environment: furniture and tools that he uses every day.

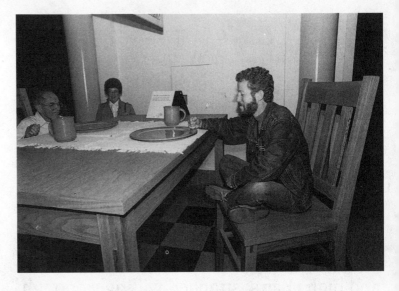

Does Your Child Need Foot Support ?

Does she:

Slump at the table?

Sit on her knees?

Sit with her knees up?

Wiggle and squirm constantly?

Spill food and knock things over?

Rush away as soon as she can?

Support herself on her elbows?

Have trouble writing neatly?

Prefer working on the floor?

If you answered yes to any of these questions, consider getting your child a chair that supports her feet.

Remember how it felt to be three years old in an adult-size world?

If he must struggle to reach things, he will be clumsy and awkward. If he is forced to use flimsy, toylike furniture, he will become sloppy and careless.

If your child must depend on you to find a toy, coat or pair of boots, if he cannot touch anything in the kitchen without your help, if books, recordings and art materials are stored out of his reach, he will remain dependent on you for years. Children become independent through a series of small discoveries: "I can dress myself, make my bed, pack my lunch, help myself to a snack." Your child cannot learn independence if common household items become a source of frustration.

The independent child becomes more capable and helpful. With each new discovery he is included in new activities around the house. Ergonomics enables a child to take the crucial steps that separate childhood from the adult world sooner and with greater ease.

This section of the book presents a child's-eye view of the home. Common objects that you take for granted present unexpected ergonomic challenges to a child. An ergonomic environment should be benevolent, even helpful, and not challenging. Plan a child-friendly home room-by-room and consider each item your

Courtesy "Sizes" exhibit, Field Museum of Natural History, Chicago, Illinois

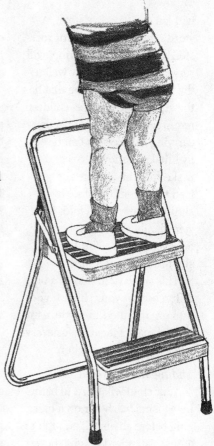

The Child's Step Stool

Once you've explained the safety issues in the kitchen—such as the dangers of knives, stove burners and scalding water—your child can enjoy helping with daily chores. Children are fascinated by the array of kitchen tools and utensils. You can count on your child to want to reach things on countertops and at cabinet height. If you don't consider his ergonomic needs, he will stand on drawers, arms of kitchen chairs, bar stools and shelves. Remember, the aim of ergonomics is to adapt the working environment to the needs of the human being, in this case a small human being. Adding the right kind of stool makes it possible for your child to work with you in the kitchen.

Don't confuse a step stool

child will use from his point of view. Focus on the qualities the item must have to make a child independent. Look closely at the tools your child depends upon daily in the home: clothing hangers, handles, drawers, personal mail, sink, shower head and stool.

Children are unable to control most adult-size tools. What's ergonomic for us—say, a regular glass or a long-handled broom, might be terribly awkward for a five-year-old. Your child shouldn't have to struggle to hang up his hat. He shouldn't be frightened by utensils that slip through his fingers and shatter on the floor. Be prepared, in the pages that follow, to rethink the tools you may have taken for granted most of your life.

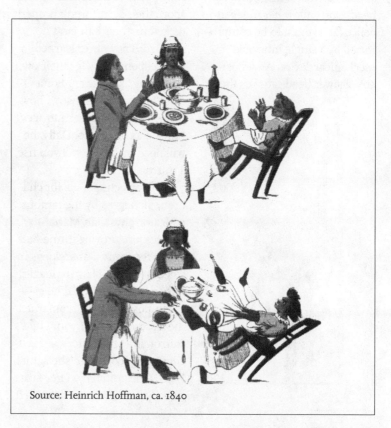

Source: Heinrich Hoffman, ca. 1840

29

with an ordinary bar stool. A sturdy step stool, made for rock-steady standing, not sitting, will serve your whole family well in the kitchen. Choose one that has the ergonomic features children require. First, the stool needs a carrying handle so it can be easily lifted and moved. Second, make sure the feet are rubberized to prevent the stool from shifting under your child. Each step should also be rubberized or covered with a similar non-slip textured material.

This small item makes a big difference for your child. It goes into use minutes after you set it up and makes it easier for everyone to relax in the kitchen.

Sliding Shower Head

Your child will learn to bathe herself and wash her own hair long before she is tall enough to adjust a standard-height shower head. Don't allow her independence (and yours) to be compromised by a single inflexible mechanical device. An adjustable shower head satisfies the

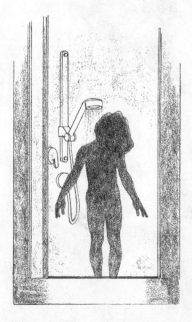

ergonomic needs of adults and children and makes the bathroom a friendlier place for everyone.

The head slides vertically on a long rod and tightens into place at any height (see illustration). Spray density and direction can then be controlled at the head by the child herself. The head-mounted control also prevents your child from getting blasted in the face. Be sure to set the water heater low enough so your child cannot accidentally scald herself. Then, turn her loose for an easy-to-control shower that's lots of fun.

The Child's Mirror

You want your child to learn to dress himself, comb his hair and look neat.

We all recognize people who grew up without these essential skills: their pants are always too short, their shirts aren't properly tucked in, their hair isn't combed. They never learned to take responsibility for their own grooming as children. For a child to develop a sense of how he looks, he must learn to see himself as others do. Daily, he will need the same tool you use, a mirror.

Self-correcting tools for children, pioneered by the famous educator-physician Maria Montessori, provide immediate tactile feedback. Square pegs in a geometrically shaped puzzle refuse to fit into round holes—it's impossible to misconstrue the lesson. Think of your child's mirror as a straightforward self-correcting tool. Once she actually sees the smudge on her face, nobody has to tell her to wash it

off. Making the decision herself, she gains a degree of independence and freedom. Without the mirror, you have nagging and arguments, the familiar penalty for poor ergonomics in the home.

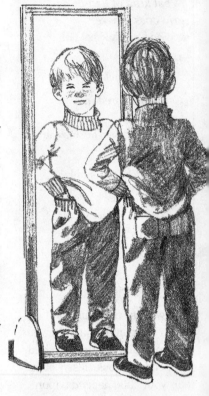

Most mirrors for adults are much too high for children to use comfortably. If your child must stand on a chair to see herself in the mirror, she'll eventually give it up; she might go through life handicapped by poor childhood ergonomics. A tiltable mirror, the ergonomic solution, will continue to provide a full body view as your child grows taller. Use shatter-proof material such as Plexiglas, if possible.

Give your children the ergonomic advantages they need to take care of themselves and they will do so.

Furniture That Grows with Your Child

All parents want their children to become independent and competent adults. But your children will only become as independent as their environment permits them to be. Away from the dining room table they need their own work surfaces and chairs as much as we do.

Avoid the common errors. Stacking two telephone books on a chair will not enable your child to magically "adapt" to adult-size furniture. Try doing calligraphy while balanced on a set of telephone books and you'll immediately understand why your child's handwriting isn't improving. Try writing a letter or reading this book at a shoulder-high desk to get a sense of the ongoing ergonomic crisis that children experience whenever they sit down to work. Most scaled-down children's furniture provides, at best, a

temporary fix, replacing a hopelessly high table with (six months later) a hopelessly low one. Either way, your child will be forced into the same awkward posture you would end up in if your table was the wrong size. And your child's work habits will be just as awkward as yours would be.

The ergonomic solution, implemented in a few preschools and fewer homes, is adjustable furniture that's made to last for years. Chair and table legs extend and then tighten into

Both the seat and foot support can be adjusted.

place to meet a child's changing requirements. Set up chairs so your child's feet rest flat on the floor while he is seated. Raise the tabletop as your child grows taller. Choose a durable work surface that's easy to clean.

The Expanding Chair

Including a child in the adult life around the dining room table teaches her many skills. She learns not just how to manage silverware and other utensils but the ceremonies that go with a meal: conversation, warmth and friendship. Banishing a child to a little table of her own sends the wrong

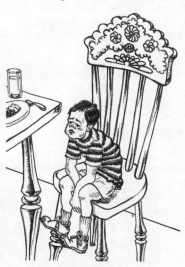

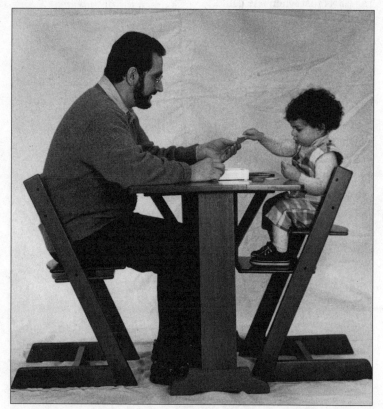

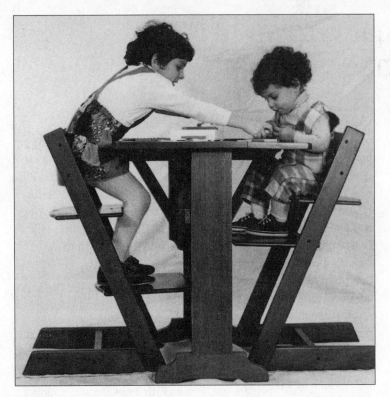

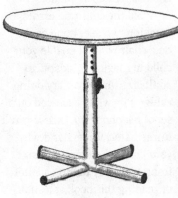

Adjustable chairs keep both children comfortable.

in his own room, where most of his mental work is done.

The fact that you can't afford new furniture every time your child grows an inch is no excuse for abandoning a child to giant chairs and tables from the ages of two to fifteen. Your child has as much right to ergonomic furniture as you do. In fact, he cannot work properly without it. The solution is furniture that's geared to the needs of your child's *growing* body: personal desks and group tables with adjustable legs. Such furniture

message: just when she could be learning table manners, she's excluded.

In order to eat and work on an adult-size table, a child needs an adjustable chair. Look for two essential adjustments: seat and footrest height. Chairs in which only the seat will move bring the child up to the table only to leave her feet dangling, a cruel joke. Avoid flimsy, toylike children's furniture; a small child should be able to keep the same chair for many years. Start her off with both the seat and footrest in the topmost position. As she grows older you can simply lower the two platforms, adjusting them to her leg and torso height. When your child's feet touch the ground, she's ready for adult furniture.

The Child-Friendly Desk

The problem your child had struggling to sit in adult-size chairs in the dining area becomes even more distracting

 The Tripp Trapp Chair
Equipment Shop
P.O. Box 33
Bedford, Massachusetts 01730
(617) 275 7681

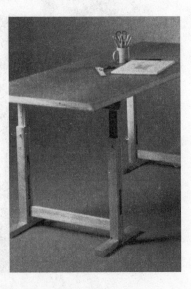

is not expensive or hard to find. Choose a sturdy table with a hard, washable surface that will double as a desk or workbench.

IKEA
20700 South Avalon Blvd.
Carson, California 90746
(310) 527 4532

Kids in the Kitchen

Bad ergonomics creates mental as well as physical problems for everyone. Do you find yourself stumbling over toys in the kitchen, spilling coffee on drawings? Do you and your child have petty arguments over missing puzzle pieces and math papers? Has your kitchen become a battleground between you and your children?

Don't waste time trying to fix the blame on other family members; you are all the victims of a massive ergonomic failure. Consider these indisputable facts of twentieth-century kitchen life: young children spend a great deal of time playing near whichever parent happens to be cooking. They will bring toys and coloring supplies and little pots and pans. As they grow older, they will spread out their homework on nearby tables—*and they have a perfect right to do so.*

Think of kitchen toys as children's tools, not clutter. If we set up the kitchen as though all play and homework must go on elsewhere, we are in full denial about the room's actual function. The social center of the home can become a tense and argumentative place.

The tools—small toys, art supplies and homework materials—that your children use in the kitchen require local storage space. You can negotiate the space requirements, drawing the line perhaps at a crayon set, a few pencils, a pad of paper and a handful of toys. Once you've provided a storage spot (say, a couple of open shelves), your children will enjoy organizing their possessions. Peace descends on your kitchen when you make room for your children's toys.

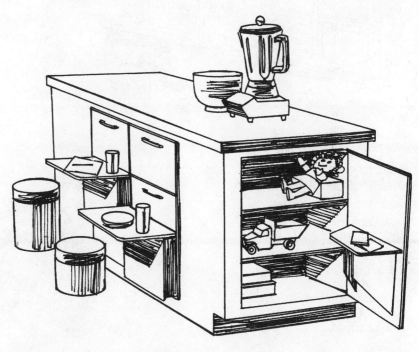

Toy Storage

Children like to keep things orderly. Too often, however, they are prevented from doing so by appalling ergonomic conditions that are imposed on them by adults. Consider the beloved toy chest, the adult-furnished storage system that children are expected to use. Cute as it is, the toy chest is simply a large box into which toys must be unceremoniously dumped. No

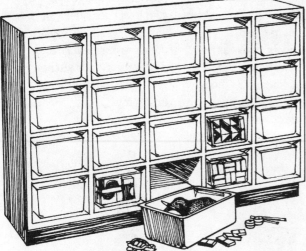

wonder chests tend to overflow and toys end up lost or broken.

Again, we are making demands on children that we wouldn't dream of making on ourselves. Would you use a desk chest to organize your office tools?

Lakeshore Learning Materials
2695 East Dominguez Street
Carson, California 90749
(800) 421 5354

Open Shelves with Transparent Storage Bins

Set up reachable storage with deep open shelves for children (see illustration). Place clear storage boxes within each shelf. Lego blocks, puzzles and toy animals are thus isolated from each other, visible and accessible. You will be amazed at how much this simple ergonomic step will mean to your child. He will play more (and watch television less) just because he can see his toys and get to them easily.

The Movable Platform

Eventually, your child will begin to combine her toys to create large, complex scenarios—a doll house and grounds, a train that passes through a Lego city, a space station made from blocks and bits of string— that she will want to preserve. Big projects, every parent learns, become big problems, even safety hazards, if you leave them set up in the middle of your living room. Cleaning becomes awkward, and socializing is nearly impossible. Instead of pulling your child's creations apart at the end of the day, provide her with an ergonomic building environment.

Children's trundle beds are usually purchased to accommodate the occasional overnight

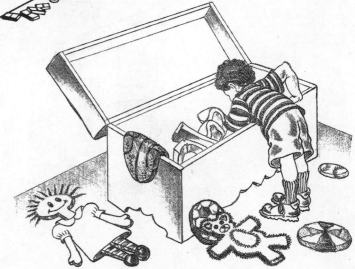

guest. If you're willing to put the little friend on an air mattress or futon for the night, you'll find that the trundle makes a generous long-term toy project platform. Mounted

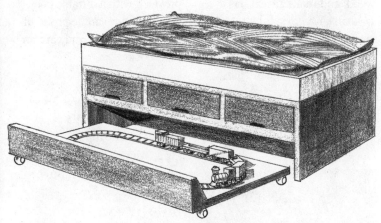

on wheels, the trundle slips beneath your child's bed effortlessly, where it stores her creations (and some spare toys) intact. If the trundle has a slatted or soft base, add a sheet of plywood to make the surface rigid enough for serious play.

The Child-Friendly Floor

Children's work is play. Just as you need space to work effectively, your children need space to play properly. Many homes are so cluttered with furniture

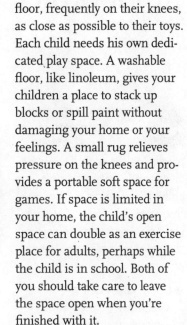

and possessions that the open space children require for play may simply not exist. The ergonomic approach is to be generous: find out how much space your children actually need and give it to them.

Young children live on the floor, frequently on their knees, as close as possible to their toys. Each child needs his own dedicated play space. A washable floor, like linoleum, gives your children a place to stack up blocks or spill paint without damaging your home or your feelings. A small rug relieves pressure on the knees and provides a portable soft space for games. If space is limited in your home, the child's open space can double as an exercise place for adults, perhaps while the child is in school. Both of you should take care to leave the space open when you're finished with it.

Having his own small rug and an open space to use it in provides a sense of personal territory, which is essential in normal development. Keeping a couple of rolled-up rugs on hand for visiting kids makes the difference between happy parallel play and fierce territorial fights.

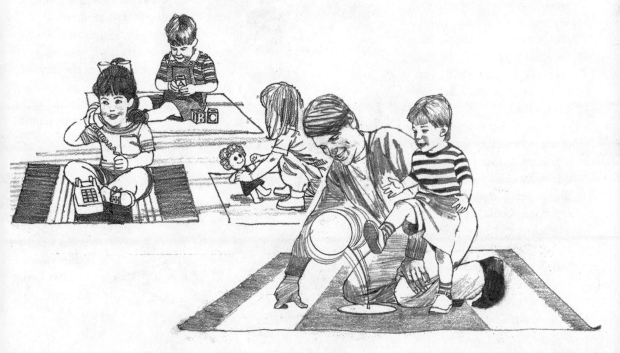

Ergonomics for Reading

Since reading is one of the most important skills your child will ever learn, his books should be visible and easily accessible. A child will revisit a favorite book frequently if it's at hand. With child-size ergonomic tools, reading becomes a pleasure instead of a chore.

A Child's Bookcase

Children's books come in whimsical sizes designed to attract and hold a beginning reader's attention. Some are extra tall, others unfold into fantastic scenarios and still others are shaped for tiny hands or disguised as little animals. All these glossy, colorful books are easy for a child to handle but difficult for adults, much less inexperienced children, to store. Without an ergonomic storage plan, the more books you buy, the greater the likelihood that every volume your child owns will end the day piled in a disorganized heap.

Nothing discourages a developing reader more than a chaotic reading environment. If you want your child to read, give him or her a durable, child-size ergonomic bookcase.

Shelves should be rounded and angled back so that your child can easily read the titles. Angled shelves also help to hold books firmly in place. Select a high-quality material like solid wood, and make sure it has a washable nontoxic finish. Make sure the bookcase has at least three different shelf sizes to store the wide range of children's books—oversize books on the bottom, medium-size books in the middle and small ones on top. Children, when provided with a durable bookcase that they can be proud of, will learn to value and care for their books.

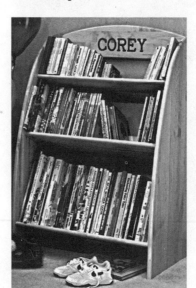

Levenger
420 Commerce Drive
Delray Beach, Florida 33445
(800) 544 0880

Texwood Furniture
3508 East First Street
Austin, Texas 78762
(512) 385 3323

A Child's Bed Lamp

A good book settles the mind at bedtime. Small children will happily imitate their parents' bedtime reading habits if you make it possible for them to do so. However, you cannot expect your child to read in bed without the same kind of ergonomic lighting that you require.

An easily adjustable wall-hung bed light with a narrow-beam spot placed at the head of your child's bed will go into use the day you set it up. Avoid tippy floor or table lamps and their precarious electrical cords. Show your child how to adjust the lamp so the light falls on her book, not in her face. Store books nearby and let your child choose a favorite title each night.

Big Art for Little Kids (and Grownups)

The smaller the child, the larger the details in his drawings. Like all art, your children's efforts are meant to be viewed and enjoyed. Little bulletin boards become clogged with layers of overlapped postings in no time. The sides of the refrigerator fill up fast. Then what? Survival of the fittest drawings? Compulsive neatness?

Commercial bulletin boards are expensive and generally too small to do justice to the out-pouring of childhood art. However, without much trouble you can create your own bulletin boards large enough to cover anything from the space above your child's desk to an entire bedroom wall. Generous bulletin boards feel good to use. Gone are the disorganized overlapping photos and drawings. Postings stand on their own. You can change the display weekly and alter the character of a whole room.

Giant bulletin boards work for adults as well. Depending on the material you choose for a covering, they provide an easy way to display posters and photos without the bother and expense of elaborate frames. You can change a display in minutes without drilling holes into the wall. Giant bulletin boards also significantly

I. Have the sound board cut to a suitable size.

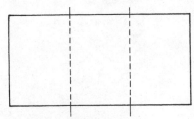

2. Cut and iron the fabric.

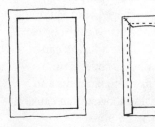

3. Staple the fabric to the sound board.

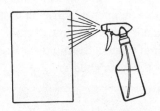

4. Spray the fabric side lightly with plain water.

improve the acoustics of a room, an important ergonomic consideration in spaces where you plan to listen to music.

Making the Board

The bulletin board material, available in four-by-eight-foot sheets at any lumber yard, is generally called *sound board.* Cover it with a *coarse* cotton canvas or muslin colored to your taste. Cut your material three to four inches wider and longer than the sound board.

Iron it to remove any wrinkles. Attaching the material to the sound board works best with two people—the job goes quickly. Fold the edge of the material tightly over the edge of the sound board. Fold the corners to eliminate wrinkles before you staple each side. Staple the folded side every six inches with 3/8-inch fasteners.

Then for a tight fit, using a spray bottle dust the fabric with a light water mist. This will shrink and smooth out the material.

Place a level across the top of the board and nail it to the wall with 1 1/2-inch headless plasterboard nails (available in various colors). When hanging the board, avoid contacting the fabric with your hammer. It dents easily. Hang your art.

Danger at Home: Ergonomics and Safety

Poor ergonomics creates long- and short-term dangers, neither of which are immediately obvious. The twenty-four-hour-a-day assault on your child's body from perfectly innocent-looking objects like lights, chairs and beds might continue for months before his schoolwork begins to decline. By then your child may need medical as well as ergonomic attention.

Safety becomes an ergonomic issue in the home when familiar objects begin to create health-threatening problems for your child. We seem to recognize the fact that the home is a deceptively dangerous place for children only during infancy. We place gates at the top of stairs, fit cabinets with safety latches and insert plastic covers into electrical outlets. Well before the child starts school, however, we abandon the clunky safety devices, the "child-proofing," and launch the youngster, unprotected, into the adult world.

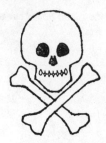

European appliance manufacturers recognize that icons and color are universally understood, language is not. But in the United States controls that might confuse an adult can easily injure a child. Round knobs in sinks, bathtubs and (especially) showers can cause a child to scald himself. Use colored tape to color code hot (red) and cold (blue) water at every faucet and replace all knobs with levers. Mark a skull and crossbones on toxics and store them on a high shelf (not under a sink) well out of children's reach. Explain the symbols to your children.

Remember: children act fast. Set up your home so your children aren't expected to navigate through a maze of loose wires or to decipher bewildering controls. Loose electrical cords can easily trip a child and bring a television down on top of him. Replace door knobs with levers that are much easier to operate with small hands. An adult carrying a child will be able to open a lever-operated door with an elbow, if necessary. Stove-top burners must be controlled with locking knobs, mounted preferably on the *side* of the cooking area (see p. 54).

Hopelessly cramped stairs, one of the most common ergonomic failures in the home, cause more accidents than all the other problems combined. Adults struggle to fit their feet onto stingy little steps, but children can end up going down a flight of stairs head first. If your stairs are particularly steep or have no landing, install a separate handrail within your child's reach.

A Child's Garden

If bad ergonomics slows down adults, it stops children cold. The garden can be nothing more than a big sandbox for your children, or it can provide one of life's great educational experiences: learning to grow food and create beauty. Her progress, indeed her very interest in the subject of gardening, is entirely dependent on ergonomics; if you provide her with the tools to grow things, she will. Make the garden a real place for your child and let her exercise her rich fantasy life elsewhere.

Children's garden tools, once little more than flimsy toys, have become as sturdy and reliable as their adult-size counterparts. Little shovels, geared to a child's height and strength, penetrate the earth. Tiny rakes gather weeds and leaves, pitchforks turn the soil and small hand tools work as well as yours for planting seedlings. Everything operates on a smaller scale, which is exactly as it should be. With the right tools your child can take responsibility for her own small plot.

Set your child up so she can complete a growing season. Dedicate a few square feet, even a window box, to her efforts. Gardening gloves, now available in children's sizes, help protect your child's hands and make the work more enjoyable.

Teach her to clean her tools after each use and provide a dedicated storage space with low pegs and shelves, ideally in your own tool shed. A set of clean, organized tools plus a selection of seeds will make your child a proud gardener. Her memory for details like the

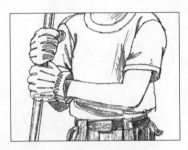

names of plants and insects is probably much better than yours. Every day her world expands in the garden. When she's big enough to use adult-size tools, she'll be ready to help with a full-size garden.

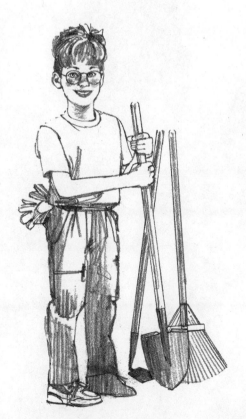

3. How to Prepare Food

When people live in one room, the hearth is generally the focal point of all activity. One enters the hut, igloo, teepee or yurt to find one's family gathered around a central cooking area. What we call kitchen work is entirely public. ❦ In Victorian times, when servants were plentiful and cheap, the kitchen was private and specialized. Physical work, relegated as much as possible to the lower classes, became an embarrassment in the bourgeois home. The social act of cooking was banished to a dark, rear kitchen where servants could come and go unseen. Food preparation went on in complete isolation from the rest of the house. ❦ The modern kitchen seems determined to burst at the seams in order to liberate its clandestine Victorian predecessor.

Kitchen Ergonomics

The Kitchen as Theater

These days the first remodeling dollars are spent demolishing walls that separate the kitchen from the space where the dining and living rooms have already merged. The "open kitchen," with its sunlit, soaring ceilings, greenhouse windows, aquariums, polished granite islands, hand-painted tiles, ubiquitous electrical devices, glittering cutlery and racks of copper pots, is celebrated in movies, architectural magazines and designer showrooms. Success means watching the soufflé rise as you relax on your sofa.

The open kitchen seems like such a generous and friendly place. Guests exchange witticisms with the affable cook, who sautés vegetables, a half-full wine glass in one hand, a spatula in the other. Subtle music tinkles away; the fireplace glows invitingly. But you, dear reader, will be the cook in your own home, not the guest reclining by the tempting hearth. You will need comfortable shoes because you will be spending plenty of

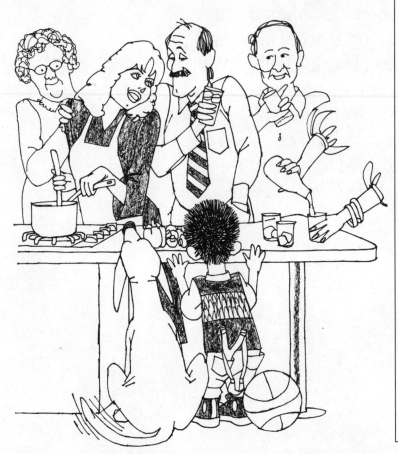

time on your feet. Eventually, most guests will gravitate to your open kitchen, where they will crowd around the stove to study your working habits. You will be the main act, perhaps the entire evening's entertainment, in your home's most demanding room.

Preparation begins long before the guests arrive. You will need to plan an appropriate stage set: attractive, orderly and clean enough to entertain anyone from your mother-in-law to your boss. Then, it's show time.

Tipsy guests, panting dogs and starving children will count on you to be polite, calm, efficient, organized, self-confident and unflappable. You will be expected to serve drinks, take urgent phone calls, make a sauce and carry on several intelligent conversations while looking after your children, who will naturally want to play at your feet. An amazing number of people carry this off—or feel they should. If you can do it and enjoy yourself, tear down those walls, build the open kitchen and equip it with ergonomic tools. But if tearful arguments erupt just before the guests arrive, don't blame your spouse—blame your surroundings. You need to make fundamental changes so your kitchen isn't doomed to become a tense and quarrelsome place, an emotional minefield at the center of your home.

> You have a right to an ergonomic kitchen in which your personal needs, both physical and mental, come first.

If you get nervous trying to socialize while you cook, you will never be happy in an open kitchen. You have a right to your own kitchen style, which can range from completely private to totally open. Compromise is possible too; a kitchen can be open for daily family meals and be closed fully or partly for entertaining. Ideally, a kitchen should give you a choice—one day it could be open, the next completely private. Choose your style, then think about specific ergonomic solutions. Never try to adapt yourself to a style that doesn't suit you.

This chapter provides ergonomic solutions for a range of kitchen layouts, all of which can be either private or completely open.

The Essential Workplace

In the kitchen bad ergonomics has been institutionalized and nailed to the floor. Doors, counters, shelves, drawers and cabinets —indeed entire sections of the room—are set up to service appliances instead of human beings.

Appliances seem intentionally designed to frustrate the people who must use them several times a day. If the electric stove required an instruction manual to do much more than fry eggs, the microwave (which is supposed to save time) directs us to read a book on "microwave cooking." The dishwasher and refrigerator have their own complex programs; most of us simply default to the basic level. As usual, each gadget demands our attention, usually while we're in a hurry to get dinner on the table.[1]

On one level the kitchen has become a kind of giant digital wristwatch, containing far too many features for anyone to bother learning. And the appliances have an arrogant quality—as though it took a gyroscope or a buzz saw to prepare food. The most elementary automated tasks—grinding coffee, beating eggs—create deafening

Open or close this kitchen according to your mood.

noise. "Nobody here but us machines." But the kitchen also remains stuck firmly in the mid-nineteenth century, with rows of cramped cabinets and counters set resolutely at the wrong height for just about everyone.

Your kitchen may have such poor ergonomics that you need to rebuild it to make a significant difference. Happily, since the kitchen is the most frequently remodeled room, you can probably expect a second chance, an opportunity to correct major ergonomic errors. When the time comes, consider the real purpose of your kitchen: it's a work space, not a decorator's fantasy. Before you consider what kind of impression your new kitchen will make, before you shop for imported tiles and sets of copper pots, consider how the kitchen itself can make your work easier.

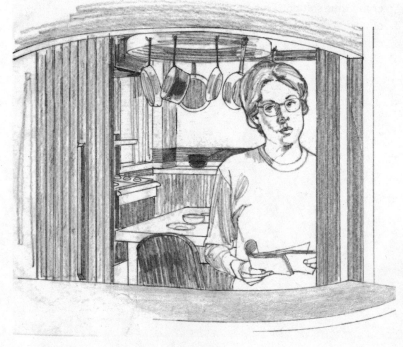

1. Similar techno-onslaughts are in progress in the living room and automobile. In the car, we're expected to program the tiny controls on digital telephones and stereos with one hand (and one eye?) while driving with the other.

Most kitchens work you too hard. Ergonomic remodeling aims to reduce the number of steps you must take, the amount of deep bending and high reaching you must do, and the accidents that occur bumping into others. You shouldn't feel as though you have walked for miles when you cook or clean. You need heat-proof materials around your stove and waterproof materials around your sink. All surfaces should be easy to clean, and tiny cracks that can collect crumbs and water and attract insect pests must be eliminated. As you will see, these little problems add up and cost you dearly.

Kitchen size matters much less than the layout of the three essential work centers: the cooktop, which includes the oven; the sink; and the food storage area, which includes the refrigerator and pantry.

The suggestions that follow show you how to evaluate your own kitchen and make the necessary ergonomic improvements.

The kitchen as suitcase

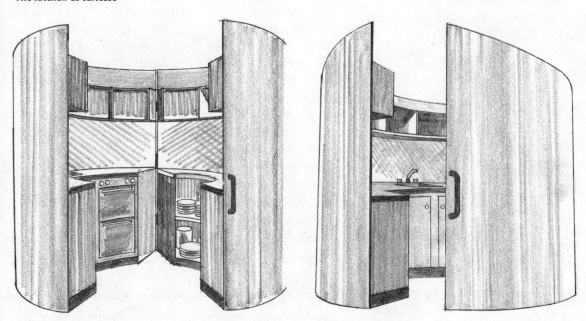

How Kitchen Floor Plans Affect You

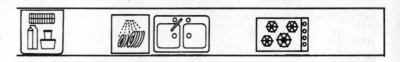

The layout of your work centers and the placement of your eating area will determine the distances you must cover in the kitchen. The logic of your storage system determines the number of trips you will make. For everyday meals, all the tools and ingredients you will need should be stored so that you can avoid high reaching or uncomfortable bending as much as possible.

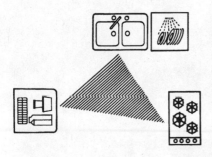

The Strip Kitchen

Strip kitchens are popular because they take up so little space. All three work centers are lined up in a straight row—a neat, if not ergonomic, approach. Traditionally, the strip was too long, stretching from one end of a rambling old ranch kitchen to the other. Now it's usually too short. Any way you set it up, however, you will end up pacing back and forth because no work triangle exists. Reducing the size of the strip, a common "solution" in efficiency apartments, cuts your overhead storage and leaves you with an insufficient countertop for food preparation.

If you're setting up a strip kitchen, observe these ergonomic guidelines:

Make sure the sink, the most frequently used work center, is in the middle.

Set up the refrigerator to open away from the counter.

Install a cushioned mat the length of the strip. It makes all the walking easier.

Space permitting, create an additional temporary workspace by adding a roll-away island.

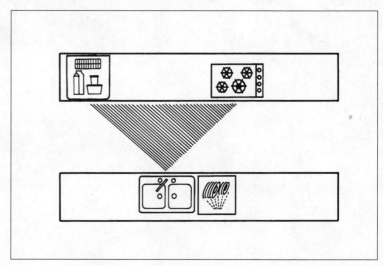

The work triangle (above), and the Pullman kitchen (right).

The Pullman Kitchen

The Pullman layout, derived from train kitchens, divides the work centers on parallel counters, a significant ergonomic improvement. As soon as one work center faces the two others, the essential work triangle begins to function. However, the corridor created by the parallel counters encourages foot traffic right through the center of the work triangle where you must manipulate hot pots and sharp knives. If one kitchen door opens to the outside, the precious work triangle can turn into an indoor freeway cluttered with discarded toys and lunch boxes.

Observe these ergonomic guidelines when setting up a Pullman kitchen:

First, try this: Bend down to take a pan out of the oven. If you hit the other side of the kitchen or bang into another person, your counters are too close to each other.

Separate the counters by at least four feet. Anything less than that will make it difficult for two people to work together in the kitchen without colliding.

While you cook, set up a barrier at one end of the kitchen. Close a door or use a movable screen.

Place rubber-backed fabric mats at each end of the Pullman corridor to catch dirt from foot traffic.

The L-shaped Kitchen

At its best, an L-shaped kitchen provides a satisfyingly compact work triangle without taking up too much floor space. The L-shape can easily become a room divider or expand to include a high counter for meals. Set up next to your major work centers, a high counter reduces the time you will spend setting the table, serving food and clearing dishes. It also provides a handy clutter barrier. People on the opposite side in, say, a dining, family or living room aren't confronted with piles of dirty dishes.

The L shape with an expanded, raised counter also directs traffic away from the work triangle. This is an effective, ergonomic kitchen design with just one potential flaw: over-extension. If the sides of the L are too long the work triangle becomes too large and you will end up with sore feet after a cooking session. Either a movable or fixed island will significantly reduce the amount of walking you need to do.

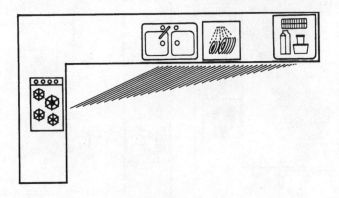

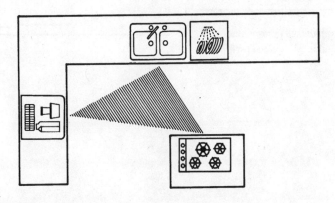

The L-shaped kitchen (above), and with the addition of an island (below).

The U-shaped kitchen

This generous layout provides the most ergonomic kitchen environment, especially if you like to cook with other people. It combines ample work surfaces with a compact work triangle—not an architectural fantasy but a work-defined space (see illustration). With the addition of an island it can accommodate a double work triangle for team cooking. The U-shaped layout can be self-contained or extend in virtually any direction to create a combination dining and family room. It functions superbly as a self-contained kitchen and also works well with room dividers. The two corner cabinets, with their deep, dark interiors, present a minor storage challenge that is easily corrected with sturdy swing-out shelves.

You can feel the difference when cooking in a U-shaped kitchen. You're walking noticeably less, and everything you need seems to be at hand.

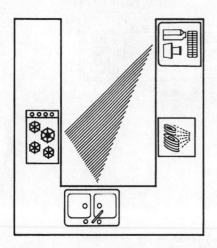 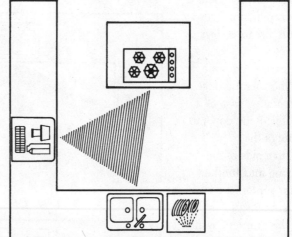

The U-shaped kitchen (above), and with the addition of an island (right).

How Effective *Is* Your Kitchen?

Make and serve a simple meal such as an ordinary breakfast. Don't change anything you usually do. Simply observe yourself closely while you work.

Notice each motion—each trip, reach, bend and stretch you must perform to make this meal:

Make juice. Get frozen juice. Get a jug. Get a long-handled spoon. Mix the juice and water. Get glasses. Set the glasses on a counter or table. Pour in the juice.

Make coffee. Get the water. Pour it in the coffeemaker. Get the coffee. Put the filter in the coffeemaker. Turn on the coffeemaker. Get cups. Pour cream and coffee.

Serve dry cereal. Get bowls and spoons. Set bowls, spoons and napkins on your table or counter. Get the cereal. Pour the cereal. Get the milk. Pour the milk.

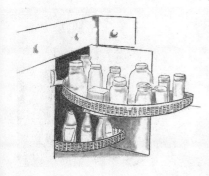

The Kitchen Test

Do you make many trips between the work centers?

Are you walking too far to get things?

Do you bump into furniture or other family members?

Are you reaching and bending all the time?

Are things hard to find?

Are you often tired and frustrated in the kitchen?

Do others have trouble managing in your kitchen?

Do houseguests find it difficult to make their own breakfast?

Can adults, children or pets snag an electrical cord and spill the contents of coffeemakers, toasters and juicers?

If the answer to any of these questions is **yes**, you need to rethink your kitchen ergonomics. You're walking too much, and the layout of your work centers is awkward. The distance to your eating area may also be too great.

Clean up and *put away* everything.

As you observe yourself, what seems like a simple operation, making breakfast, becomes a complex maneuver. Once you break your work down into individual tasks, you can see for yourself how bad ergonomics costs you dearly. Each task exacts its penalty in time and fatigue.

Kitchen errors that will drive you mad:

A refrigerator door that opens in the wrong direction

An entrance door that collides with another door

A pullout cutting board that blocks a utensil drawer

Heavy traffic through your work center

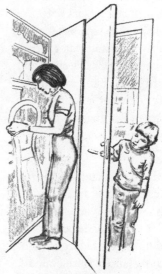

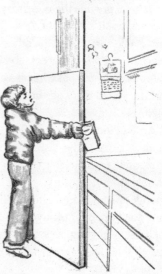

Work Centers: The Kitchen Sink

A kind of controlled chaos prevails around the main work center—the kitchen sink. Tools, food scraps and assorted junk seem to accumulate endlessly on the nearby countertops. Kitchen maintenance involves bizarre, meaningless routines in which dozens of little items are moved from one pile to another. Stacks of utensils and china teeter perilously, cups and plates turn up with inexplicable chips and weird smells hang over the sink no matter how often it is cleaned. Nothing seems to work smoothly.

Sink Clutter

If you're having trouble managing large pots and pans and cannot replace your sink with a much larger model, consider adding a spray fixture or high arching faucet. The elevated faucet will provide the necessary space to wash a deep pot. A retractable spray hose, the other alternative, gives you access to the interior of the pot while permitting you to rinse off the sink itself.

Among the new tools in the modern kitchen, the cleaning implements tend to collect in a jumble around the sink. Sponges begin to mold rapidly if they don't dry out quickly after each use. Rubber gloves slip into the sink, where they fill with water. Brushes and soaps also end up in the sink, where they grow moldy and start to smell.

A ventilated tilt-out shelf under the sink provides the crucial storage space for rubber gloves and sink cleanup tools. Hang specialized cleaning tools from a rack over the sink. Adding a pump-operated soap dispenser to the sink top further reduces clutter and allows one-handed dish soaping.

All cooking produces food scraps that ideally should go directly into the sink. If, however, the sink edge is elevated, the sweeping process will be interrupted by dirt-catching edges. A countertop made of a material like Corian or Formica 2000, thick plastic sheets that can be cut to shape, will accept a bottom-mounted sink. The top lip of the sink is fastened and sealed to the bottom of the counter, creating a water-tight transition from countertop to sink bottom, a significant ergonomic advantage.

If you discover chipped glasses and cracked plates too often in your sink, insert a rubber mat to soften the bottom of the sink. The mat also reduces the tendency of cast-iron pots to scratch the sink.

Avoid round knobs in all your sinks. Both children and elderly people have trouble operating

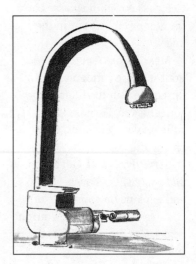

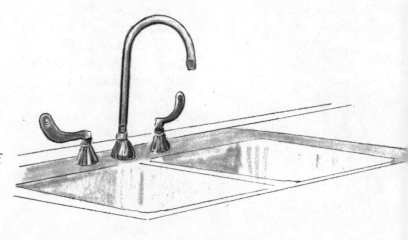

them, as will anyone with soapy hands. Substitute lever-type handles that can be grasped easily.

The fact that small children enjoy unloading dishwashers and sorting silverware points up a fundamental ergonomic problem: dishwashers are mounted much too low. Elevating your dishwasher, even six inches, will make a major difference. A low countertop dishwasher provides a truly ergonomic solution.

Are you interrupted frequently at the kitchen sink? If you have an artist in the family who needs to wash brushes, a gardener who wants to water plants and a second cook who wants to wash vegetables, you need a second sink. Set up the second sink to meet the needs of your other family members (higher for adults, lower for children). Use an island if possible.

If clean items pile up on counters around the sink, forming hazardous mountains of utensils and china, rethink your nearby storage. Your immediate storage plan around the sink should be designed to eliminate extra steps whenever possible. Store everyday items like coffee mugs, cereal bowls and knives within easy reach of your cleanup center. A magnetic strip fastened to the wall keeps your knives visible and handy. To dry and store larger utensils, hang them on their own storage rack.

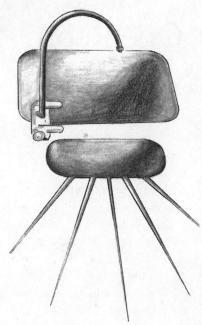

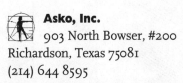

Seamless sink with built-in drain board

The Drain Board

The little ergonomic insults sting the worst. The tiny crack between your sink and the counter seems to soak up water every time you wash a dish. You sponge at it routinely, but the counter stays wet. Somehow, water seems to flow backwards from the crack onto the countertop. Tiny food particles lodge there; insects appear late at night.

We are in denial about our dish-washing habits. The time has come to eliminate needless kitchen work by combining the sink and drain board. A few manufacturers have already managed to merge the two in a single seamless unit. Water cannot collect anywhere but in the sink.

Asko, Inc.
903 North Bowser, #200
Richardson, Texas 75081
(214) 644 8595

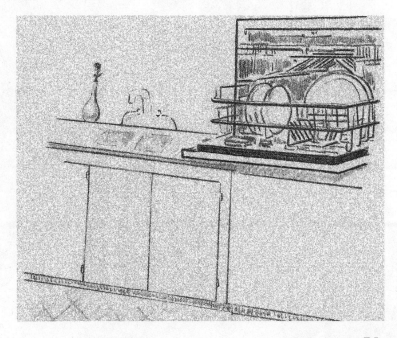

Many Cooks, One Room

Most kitchens are not set up to accommodate more than one cook at a time. Yes, with extra courtesy, coordination and balance, two cooks can manage to coexist in one room, but the dedicated two-cook kitchen makes the social engineering unnecessary. If you're a fan of team cooking, consider installing an extra sink in your kitchen. You have to experience the difference this small ergonomic feature makes to believe it.

Each cook not only needs his own sink, he must be able to work as though he were the only cook in the kitchen. Placement of the sinks is critical to making the kitchen function equally well for both. Each sink should be on the outside edge of two independent triangular work spaces (see diagram). You can use facing counters or set up one of the sinks on an independent island.

Each cook should also have his own countertop. Install counters to accommodate each individual's height. If you have space for an island, use it to set up a second counter next to the second sink. Again, no matter which configuration you choose, to avoid collisions between two cooks, be sure your work centers do not overlap. The second, smaller sink complements the main double sink, which provides the necessary space for major cleanups. Use the small sink for rinsing food.

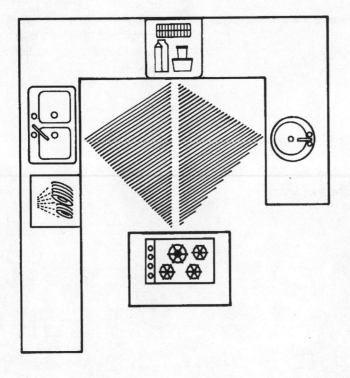

The Cooktop

Since most kitchen work takes place around the stove, it can easily become the warmest, dirtiest and most polluted place in the home. You simply cannot afford to let a task as important as food preparation turn into an unpleasant ordeal. You have ergonomic choices in the kitchen that didn't exist a few years ago.

Open gas burners admit black sludge that collects on the shelf below, where it clings to delicate internal gas lines and controls. Whenever food can get under a burner, it will, you can depend on it. The longer you put off the wearisome cleaning job, the worse it gets.

Sealed gas burners completely eliminate this tedious job. Put them at the top of your list when you remodel your kitchen.

Vents

Stove manufacturers love to ignore the laws of physics. Where there's fire, there's smoke; sometimes it's visible, sometimes not. You shouldn't have to pollute your living space to cook dinner, but that's what you'll end up doing if you don't remove stove exhaust from your kitchen. The carbon monoxide produced by open gas flames is colorless and odorless. Small

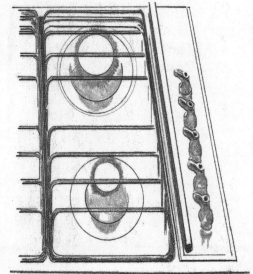

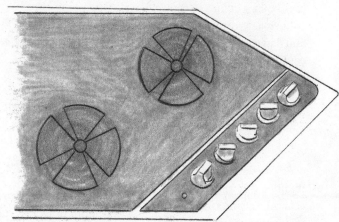

Sealed gas burners (left), and safe cooktop controls (below). Smoke is sucked down and blown away (bottom).

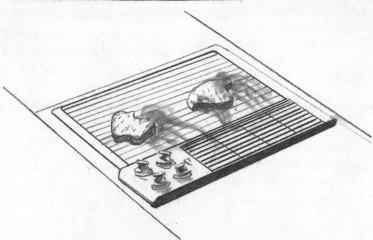

doses can give you a headache and make you irritable. We all know what larger doses do.

Make sure your stove is vented to the outside, either with a top-fitting hood or, if that's impractical, a down-venting system that can draw exhaust gases through the floor if necessary. Keep exhaust fans well oiled and comfortably quiet.

Controls

Stove controls once were the main ergonomic trouble spot in the kitchen until the microwave oven arrived. The typical setup, a row of six identical rotary buttons that controls four burners, a griddle and an oven, will have you thinking twice about how to boil water five years after you buy the stove. Furthermore, the buttons, which are generally placed along the front lip of the stove, become a powerful temptation to children. Make absolutely sure that your burner controls have a "childproofing" mechanism that requires the burner to be pushed in before it can be rotated. Stoves with burner controls on the back splash panel simply substitute one safety hazard for another. Reaching over boiling liquids to control your stove is obviously awkward and dangerous. Childproofed controls mounted along the side of the burners offer a practical ergonomic compromise.

Traditional Ovens

To save space, millions of stoves are built with stovetops over knee-level ovens. This traditional arrangement, while economical and compact, has major ergonomic drawbacks. It forces you to bend down to check on food while a rush of humid, superheated air blasts you right in the face. If you wear glasses, you may be temporarily blinded by the hot mist. Furthermore, you will be expected to extract heavy, hot dishes from an underlighted compartment near the floor. Yes, you can manage it most of

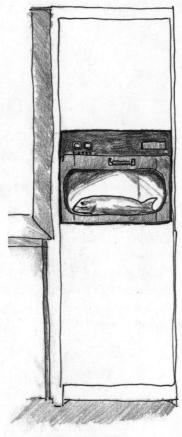

Well-lighted, chest-high oven

the time, but this is precisely the kind of hopeless ergonomics that puts people in the emergency room.

When you remodel or choose a new kitchen, reject the traditional stove-oven configuration in favor of a completely separate oven, mounted chest high, which permits you to manipulate and view heavy loads much more easily. You will experience the ergonomic advantages the first time you cook. A good oven also requires a large safety-glass door and a brightly lighted interior, so you can check on food without letting the heat escape (or the cake collapse). Despite the popularity of safety-glass doors, many ovens remain

underlighted, making them difficult, even dangerous, at any height. Check the interior lighting before you buy an oven.

Microwave Ovens

The microwave oven has one of the most hopeless user interfaces of any household appliance. Faced with a daunting, twenty-button keypad and a fifty-page manual, most people never advance beyond learning to cook potatoes without turning them into glue. For the most part, the icons, timers and programs are simply never used. Like the programmable thermostat and the VCR, the microwave oven is seldom pushed beyond its most basic capabilities. At some point you have to say to yourself, I am an educated adult, and I'm not getting anywhere with this machine. When you confront an ergonomic failure, you realize that you're right, and the machine is wrong.

More than twenty years after its introduction, the microwave still needs to become much easier to use, or it never will fulfill its potential.

The machine is not only difficult to program, it has become a space hog. Built-in models preserve precious counter space, an ergonomic plus.

If you use a microwave only for defrosting and heating up leftovers, place the machine close to the refrigerator. If you integrate it into your general cooking scheme, put the microwave near your cooktop.

The Refrigerator

The refrigerator, now universally taken for granted, has been with us for less than a century. Like most popular innovations in the home—the VCR, the efficiency kitchen, the stereo—its ergonomics have been ignored in favor of progress (size plus gadgetry). People love refrigeration, reasoned the marketeers, so let's make it bigger and programmable (and more expensive).

Refrigerators have performed their magic for decades and since they usually do it without complaint, we've trained ourselves to endure little ergonomic insults in order to have fresh food on hand. When we're ready for a new one, we think immediately about size, color and automatic ice making. But this purchase offers you the opportunity to address, finally, some of the most crucial ergonomic issues of indoor cold storage: noise and accessibility.

Don't allow yourself to be talked into more refrigerator space than you actually need. Remember, the refrigerator is nothing more than a storage system, and without easy access to the food inside you cannot use it effectively. Simply installing a huge refrigerator should not tempt you to try to store a three-month supply of perishable food, because most of it will spoil. (A fundamental

The Refrigerator Test

Avoid bending
bottom-mounted freezer

Reduce noise
quiet motor

Easy access
slide-out shelves

Visibility
transparent compartments

Avoid spoiling
bigger isn't always better

Check footprint
space to open the door

question to ask before buying: Who will clean it?) If, however, your refrigerator is average size and your food is still constantly spoiling, consider slide-out shelves. You need better access, not more space.

For adults with no children, the most popular refrigerator design, the freezer on top, is the least ergonomic. Children, one can argue, require low access to refrigerated items. But there is no good reason for adults to store the most frequently handled foods—fruits and vegetables—in foot-level bins. The things you don't need daily, frozen items that must remain undisturbed until they are consumed, shouldn't be permitted to dominate your most accessible storage area at eye level. If you hate bending to

remove items from vegetable and fruit bins, consider a model with the freezer on the bottom. Also, look for transparent fruit and vegetable drawers that will permit you to see what you've stored, an ergonomic advantage.

Before you buy a refrigerator, listen to the compressor cycle on and off. Noise levels vary greatly.

The refrigerator's footprint, the amount of floor space it will occupy in your kitchen, must be measured with the door open. If you have trouble opening the door fully, get a double-door model with a freezer on one side and a refrigerator on the other. It's a bit more expensive to operate but much easier to organize. The shorter, more ergonomic shelves resist pileups and cramming.

The Loading Counter and the Pantry

Without a loading and unloading counter next to your refrigerator, your kitchen will become a little gymnasium where scattered grocery bags take the place of weights. Make absolutely sure your loading counter is opposite the refrigerator door hinge. A shelf on the hinge side of the door forces you to reach around the door to use it. Most refrigerators doors can be hung from either side. Adjust yours to accommodate the loading and unloading shelf.

If your family requires a separate freezer, consider a vertical model with many shelves. With or without wire baskets, the horizontal bin-type freezer ultimately becomes a three-foot-high pile of ancient food souvenirs. Only the most dedicated housekeeper will remember what's at the bottom; most of us would rather not find out. While slightly cheaper to operate, a horizontal freezer is much more difficult to manage than a vertical model.

Food Storage

You need dark dry storage (grains), dark cool storage (potatoes), and horizontal storage (wine), as well as storage for big, little and amorphously shaped things. You also need to store cans so that they don't roll around. Ideally, the pantry can be used for all of these purposes. Glassed cabinets aren't appropriate since food is best stored in darkness. Make sure that direct sunlight cannot penetrate your pantry.

A two-story lazy Susan and theater shelves

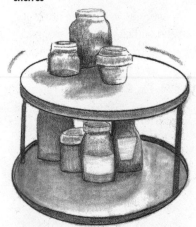

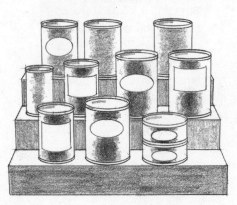

The principles of ergonomic storage throughout the kitchen also apply within the pantry. Set up an active system in which as many categories as possible are visible. Before you pack the pantry from floor to ceiling, think carefully about your cooking needs and store the most commonly used items between knee and eye level. If possible, make your pantry a walk-in space with bright interior lighting. Use door-mounted shelves, lazy Susans and theater shelves (see illustration) for small items. Store foods like bulk grains and pasta in see-through plastic containers. The refrigerator and pantry constitute one of the essential points of the work triangle; the entire kitchen will work better if you keep them close together.

Hold Everything
P.O. Box 7807
San Francisco, California 94120
(800) 421 2264

Lighting the Kitchen

The traditional large, centrally located ceiling light provides enough ambient light to eliminate shadows and dark corners. However, it cannot take care of all your lighting needs. If you have a main ceiling light, make sure the light passes through a diffused surface. If it hums or blinks, replace it.

The ergonomic challenge in the kitchen is to provide independent task lighting for each of your work centers as well as soft, pleasing light for the eating table and counter. Since kitchen eating areas double as work places for homework, sewing, art projects and other activities, you will need both kinds of lighting. Set up task lights (such as adjustable track fixtures) over every work area, and add dimmers to the lights that serve eating areas.

Lighting Ergonomics

Do:
  Use dimmers
  Use task lights over work centers
  Install reflective window shades

Don't tolerate:
  Glare
  Noisy fixtures
  Industrial lighting while eating

Generally, lights work best when installed on the ceiling. If you must use wall mounts, take extra care not to discriminate against left-handed cooks, and be sure your task lights do not create glare or shadows on the work centers. Mount a light over the center of each work area. Dark materials, like wood, require significantly more light than light materials.

Pantries, cupboards and other deep, sunless storage areas require their own lighting, which should be switched, automatically, at the door. Independently lighted ovens and refrigerators are usually taken for granted until their nonstandard bulb fails. Make sure you have extra bulbs on hand so you don't end up struggling to cook in a dark oven.

If your kitchen has south-facing windows, glare can become a major, unacknowledged problem. Don't try to get accustomed to the glare—you never will. Rather than squinting during each meal preparation, hang metal-backed translucent shades on your windows. They will reflect light and heat during the sunny hours while preserving some of your view. Glare gives way to a soft and pleasant light that transforms the kitchen. The shades also help to insulate your kitchen while preserving your privacy.

The Deafening Kitchen (and What You Can Do about It)

Each new crop of labor-saving machines helps the kitchen fulfill its role as the industrial center of the home—while raising the noise level.

Since we hate to view our homes as workplaces, we think nothing of operating deafening machines without ear protection. Hearing loss, unfortunately, is cumulative and eventually, irreversible (see p. 135). Nevertheless, the protections against noisy machinery that are routinely provided to industrial workers are blithely ignored in the home.

Typically, kitchens are the least acoustically friendly places in the home. Hard, slick, easy-to-clean surfaces bounce annoying sounds from one wall to the other. Coffee grinders, blenders and food processors that begin at ear-splitting volume seem to get louder as you use them. Refrigerators, garbage compactors and dishwashers add a low-pitched rumble capable of penetrating walls and actually shaking whole rooms. If exhaust fans are difficult to oil, most people resign themselves to the sound of dry metal bearings grinding against each other at high speeds. In fact, most kitchen noise carries far beyond the kitchen itself. Remember that if you're thinking about opening your kitchen to the living room.

Though you're expected to tolerate an infernal racket in the kitchen (it saves time!), you cannot afford to do so. Modern kitchens are perfectly capable of generating noise levels high enough to cause permanent hearing loss, especially in children. You shouldn't have to risk your two-year-old's hearing in order to make dinner. But long before real damage begins, the insidious effects of noise cause irritability, even aggression, that lasts for hours. Don't let a noisy kitchen throw an invisible monkey wrench into your best-laid plans for a relaxed evening.

Control noise whenever you can in your kitchen, never take it for granted. Apply the same sound-control measures in your kitchen that office workers use. Put all countertop machines on thick rubber pads. Since foam rubber office pads are difficult to wash, a thick rubber sink pad is more effective. Listen to new appliances before you buy them. Noise levels vary greatly, especially with dishwashers and refrigerators. Open shelves, hanging stove hoods, and tool racks will limit the tendency of irritating sounds to bounce freely. Oil ceiling, oven and microwave exhaust fans; doing so makes them significantly quieter. If you must operate a blender or juicer for long periods, say, to prepare drinks for a party, wear earplugs.

When you're ready to remodel, ignore the carpeting, hanging textiles and acoustic tiles that look so inviting in "dream kitchen" photo spreads. These materials simply don't belong in kitchens. Real sound control begins under the walls where standard thin wall construction can turn your kitchen into a giant sounding board; the walls literally vibrating in sympathy with every kitchen appliance. Build your walls with a layer of acoustically dead sound board beneath a double layer of plasterboard. This invisible and relatively inexpensive modification will make your kitchen feel like a castle with foot thick walls. Vibrations from dishwashers and refrigerators that once shook the rafters will stop at the walls.

The Storage Plan

You own it, but will you use it? Your kitchen is expected to provide space for hundreds of items, many of which have vastly different storage requirements. Various foods need to be kept cold, dry and dark in the same room.

Tools range from fragile (glass) to industrial (machines); some are sharp (knives), others toxic (lye). Without an ergonomic storage plan your tools end up hibernating in the back of forgotten cabinets. The kitchen becomes a long-term storage garage for old food and older appliances.

Anything you actually expect to use in the kitchen, whether it's animal, vegetable or mineral, must be easy to find and put back.

Hanging Storage

Hang nonmagnetic, frequently used kitchen tools from horizontal racks. Tool bars, suspended from the ceiling or attached to a wall, permit you to suspend utensils directly over your work area. To avoid crowding, a simple hanging bar will expand your storage possibilities. A tool bar will accept slotted racks for soap and small bottles as well as a variety of extension devices that permit you to hang banks of small items together.

 Hold Everything
P.O. Box 7807
San Francisco, California 94120
(800) 421 2264

Knife Storage

When you need a knife, you need it immediately. Drawers keep your knives hidden, mixed together and accessible to young children. Slotted wood blocks are difficult to clean. Hang your knives on a wall-mounted magnetic strip, well out of young children's reach, directly over your food preparation counter. A magnetic strip eliminates the intermediate drain-basket step after you wash your knives. Simply hang them up to dry.

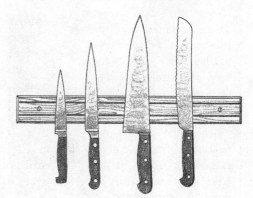

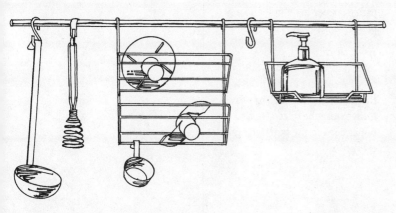

Tool bar and magnetic knife holder

Ergonomic Kitchen Storage Essentials

Proximity

Store things as close as possible to the place where they will be used. Keep pots near the stove and knives next to a food preparation counter. Items like dishes and silverware that spend time in two places—the dishwasher and the dining table—can be stored near either one.

Gadgets

If you can't put your hands on it when you need it, it's probably buried somewhere under the kitchen counter. You may never see it again.

Visibility

Open shelving provides great visibility but also becomes a dust trap. In earthquake-prone areas, open shelving becomes empty shelving sooner or later. Ideally, your cabinets should have semi-translucent (tinted, brushed or wire-impregnated) glass doors, which permit a cook to see what's inside without displaying every detail of the contents to others.

Access

Keep food in see-through containers. Install lights in deep, dark cabinets. Place spice jars and other little items on a lazy Susan or theater ramp (see p. 56).

Logic

Store things together that are used together. Juicer attachments belong next to the juicer, whisks next to the mixing bowls.

Stackables

Purchase cups, mugs, glasses and bowls for everyday use that fit together and your storage requirements will shrink by half or more. Listen for the satisfying little click when they make contact in your cabinet.

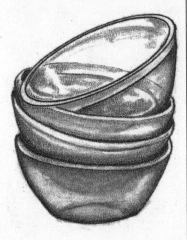

Priorities

The most valuable real estate in your kitchen is the territory you can reach from your work triangle. Save the storage space in this area for your most frequently used items: for the coffee drinker, a coffeemaker and mug; for the family with a new child, a baby bottle, a cup, a spoon, and so on; for everybody, essential knives, basic pots and pans, a paper-towel roll and a pepper mill.

Frequency

Arrange other kitchen equipment according to this principle: frequency corresponds to proximity. Store the once-a-year punchbowl in the farthest, highest cabinet.

Active Storage

Start by rethinking your storage routine—you don't have to accept your kitchen as it is. An ergonomic approach to storage, a daily task, can save you hours every week.

Begin by putting things where they are easy to reach without uncomfortable stretching and bending. Store frequently used items visibly, between knee and eye level. Open shelves, although inviting, gather dust and create extra work for you. They also become a hazard in earthquake country. Glassed cabinets provide the same visibility while eliminating an extra round of weekly cleaning. They work well in any kind of kitchen.

Appliance Garages

Large kitchen appliances have a way of disappearing after an intitial honeymoon period. You can prevent this wasteful practice by never buying anything without first having a clear idea of where you will store it. Appliance garages, built into the walls above or below the countertop, provide a permanent home for each machine.

You shouldn't have to battle your way through stacks of clattering pots and pans to get at your food processor. Like the deskbound office worker, the modern cook is deluged with space-hungry "work savers." They either dominate precious counter space or disappear completely, thus demonstrating one of the basic ergonomic kitchen truths: large machines cannot be stored effectively in ordinary drawers or, worse, deep shelves in corner cabinets. Beware of "temporary" closet solutions. Too many perfectly good appliances hibernate in dark closets forever.

Dedicated shelves that pull or swing out make your appliances a pleasure to use. Make this a high priority when you remodel or build. Whether or not you plan to remodel, you need a plan to guard invaluable countertops from mechanical clutter. If you have a little extra space in the kitchen, set up machine storage in an island or on a roll-around cart.

If you like to plan ahead you will prefer either a separate kitchen or one that can be open for small gatherings but closed for demanding productions (see p. 44). However, if you prefer to improvise, go for the completely open kitchen.

Toxic Storage

Now that the kitchen has become a social center, a gathering place for the family, your children will quite naturally want to play nearby while you cook. This should be fun, not life threatening.

Since every tool and virtually every appliance is potentially dangerous, we nag and frighten children with nasty parables about touching hot stoves. But the stakes in the kitchen are much higher than a singed fingertip. Just beneath the sink, within easy reach of children and pets, is the toxic dump of the modern home.

Don't let nasty chemicals stop you from making the kitchen into a safe and friendly place. Warning your kids doesn't protect other people's children. You wouldn't store a loaded gun behind a childproof latch; don't depend on one to protect your children from caustic liquids. Move toxics to eye-level storage, high enough to be out of a child's reach but not so high that they will fall on you as you reach for them. Never store toxic substances and foods on the same shelf.

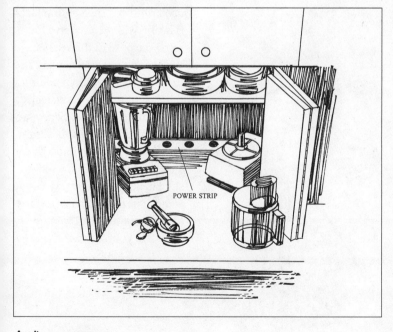

POWER STRIP

Appliance garage

Standing or Sitting

We hate to think of our home as yet another workplace. The job takes its toll on the body from nine to five, after which we try not to think about stress.

Our bodies, however, cannot choose to ignore the external world; we are as much at risk from poor ergonomics at home as in the office. Most kitchen work, for example, must be done while standing; we have no choice. By the time we learn to cook, we know by heart the slow dance of rinsing, mixing, stirring and pouring that takes us around the kitchen triangle. But the dance has pauses—peeling fruit, chopping vegetables, icing a cake—that most kitchen layouts never acknowledge. Ergonomics teaches us that the human body works better when it is not locked into a single posture. A physical change in your job description is an ergonomic opportunity. In the office we sit when we could stand; in the kitchen we stand on fatigued legs when we could easily sit.

Resist the puritanical notion that all kitchen work must be done while standing. When you get a chance to sit down, for jobs that take more than a minute or two, do so. A high chair with lumbar support and a footrest should be a permanent part of your kitchen. A drafting chair, covered with material that can be wiped clean, works well too. Make sure your kitchen contains a counter with a cut-out space for your knees where you can work comfortably while seated.

When you must stand, think about the most ergonomic way to do so. If your counters are too high or too low, add a roll-around island that's adjusted to your height. Small padded rubber mats at each work area, used routinely in standing factory work, will readily serve the same purpose in the kitchen. We spend thousands on kitchen improvements without adding this essential ergonomic tool. Standing on the mat, as any factory worker will tell you, significantly eases the strain on your legs and feet. Use a low footstool to elevate one leg while you stand. You'll be surprised at the difference this small variation makes to your lower back.

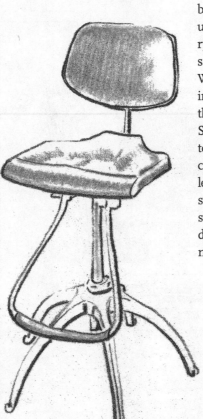

Every cook is entitled to a decent chair.

Kitchen Entertainment

Whether you listen to the morning news or practice cooking to video instructions, it's handy to have an audiovisual system in the kitchen. Finding a place to put it, however, always compromises your space requirements. You can never have enough counter space in the kitchen, and you will come to resent, possibly even damage, any audiovisual equipment that comes between you and the family dinner. If you can't give up counter space, what can you give up?

Bose Corporation
The Mountain
Framingham, MA 01701
(800) 282 2673, ext. 491

To eliminate the footprint problem, hang your set on the wall. Mount your television on a swiveling wall bracket, which will give you an unobstructed view from various parts of the kitchen. Avoid separate audio components—you won't do critical listening in the kitchen. A single-chassis unit with contained speakers works best. To eliminate a second kitchen system altogether, consider adding a set of wireless speakers, which can also hang from the wall, to your main system. They require a nearby electrical outlet.

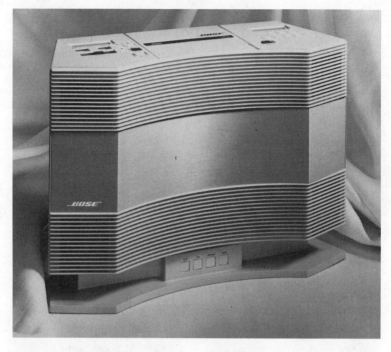

A one-piece kitchen sound system that will also play compact disks

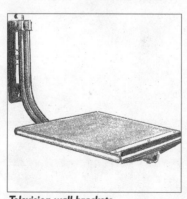

Television wall brackets

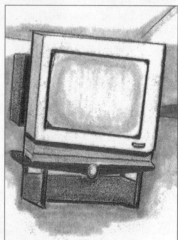

The Decline of the Family Dinner

We seem to be in denial about what goes on when we eat at home. The family dinner, during which a group ate and talked at the same table, has been widely replaced by the TV dinner, which is consumed with little or no social interaction.

Our diets vary almost as much as our schedules. One person seldom takes responsibility for everyone's meals, so we eat when we can. We're often rushed and so is our food.

Night after night we assume the familiar eating position of the late twentieth century: shoulders hunched up, knees together under a precariously balanced plate, neck bent back, eyes glued to the television screen. We've learned to hold that precarious posture for hours while the fork finds its way from plate to mouth. If our shoulders refuse to relax and our lower back goes into spasm, we swallow an extra aspirin and switch channels.

The ergonomic approach to such dining is to provide tools that serve your actual needs, not to make the process clumsy or even health threatening by denying it's happening. Eat what you like wherever you like; this is not a diet book or a religious tract.

Most dining equipment is designed for the traditional, single-table, sit-down family din-ner; it doesn't work well when we fan out to the living room or bedroom. With the appropriate ergonomic tools, however, our new dining styles begin to work more effectively. First, define your dining habits, then select your tools.

Start by accepting the way you eat. Don't change your personal habits because your dining room table looks lonely. Our dietary requirements as well as our work schedules have become more diverse; we can't always manage to be on hand when the dinner bell rings. We now understand that one individual, traditionally a woman, can't always take charge of all meal planning, shopping and cooking. And we like television with our meals. Yes, we wander in and out of the kitchen at random hours with heaping plates of food, but we've started taking responsibility for our own nourishment and cleanup. We eat when and where we feel like it.

Ergonomic Solutions for TV Dining

TV dining comes with its own set of ergonomic pitfalls. Food that's balanced on the knees is frequently spilled. Diners make multiple trips to get silverware, drinks, food and napkins. When the meal is completed, dishes become difficult and messy to manage.

Borrow a few techniques from the airline industry. Eat in an upright chair with lumbar support. Use a sturdy tray large enough for dishes and cutlery,

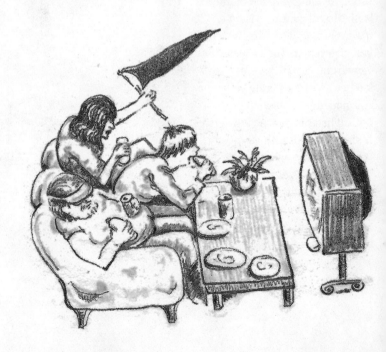

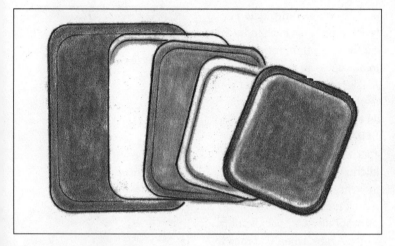

Set up a microwave (at child's height if necessary) and a snack center near the refrigerator to make browsing much easier. Store food in containers that can go directly from the refrigerator to the microwave and then to the snack counter. Browsers will want to eat out of the same bowl. Shatterproof, oven-safe glass bowls with covers work well.

and color code it for each family member. If you're resolutely married to your television at dinner time, replace the low coffee table in your living room with a long, narrow, dining-room-height table. Elevate the television, not your neck. Hanging a TV set on the wall in your formal dining room will also preserve your neck and back; however, conversation will cease the moment you release the mute button.

Browsing— Fast Food at Home

Browsers have a twofold ergonomic dilemma: where to put things and how to heat food quickly. Browsing usually takes place at the refrigerator, where food is consumed cold as the browser stands. It would taste better hot, but that seems complicated. Browsers don't plan or schedule.

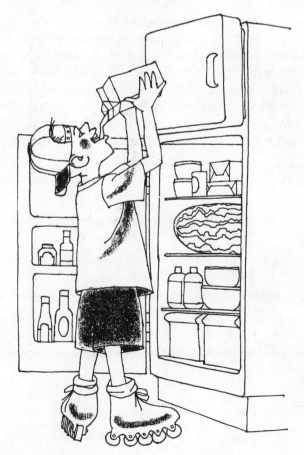

Kitchen Snobbery and Ergonomics

Design magazines promote opulent kitchens that are meant to impress visitors to your home. Happily, it's beyond the scope of this book to fiddle with anyone's interior decorating scheme. Go right ahead and hang bushels of copper pots from every rafter, install stained glass windows, suspend tropical plants from little brass hooks or build a space-age kitchen with mirrored walls and thirty-foot ceilings. But remember: style has nothing to do with ergonomics. Down-home country can work as well in the kitchen as high-tech minimalism.

Since the kitchen is the main work center in your home, you simply cannot afford to ignore ergonomic principles here. Take care of essential kitchen ergonomics first, then decorate to taste. Don't be intimidated by lavish scenarios. A plain kitchen can be very ergonomic and a joy to use while an awe-inspiring "designer" kitchen can set your teeth on edge every time you fry an egg.

Readers who live in small apartments should realize that a kitchen doesn't have to be large to be ergonomic. In fact, in large rooms it becomes difficult to incorporate a compact work triangle. Again, when it comes to equipping your kitchen, more is often less. Paring kitchen equipment down to high-quality, hardworking essentials is the most effective and ergonomic approach. Although many ergonomic solutions for the kitchen can involve costly remodeling, all of the quick fixes listed here make a significant difference.

Kitchen Ergonomics

Quick-fix solutions

Footstool
Step stool
Utensil racks
Magnetic knife strip
Lazy Susan
Theater stand
Rubber mats for standing
Appliance mats for soundproofing
See-through food storage containers
Bright lights in pantry
A roll-around island
TV dinner trays
Television on wall-mounted bracket
Ergonomic knife handles

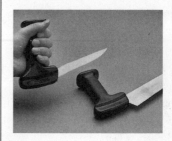

Wireless speakers
Stackable glasses, bowls and cups
Dimmers on ambient light sources
Recycling bins with handles

AliMed
297 High Street
Dedham, Massachusetts 02026
(800) 225 2610

4. How to Relax

Archaeologists will someday conclude that the main purpose of the American home in the closing years of the twentieth century was watching television. On average, we spend five hours a day watching other people telling us what to buy, and then we rush out and buy it. Happily, it's beyond the scope of this book to deliver a sermon on materialism. We must, however, address the ergonomic question: where do we put the stuff when we get it home? ❧ The fight for human dignity and freedom doesn't only happen in novels; it happens in the living room, where we battle daily with our own insatiable desire for giant closets. ❧ You don't deserve to be tormented by your own hard-won possessions.

Your Stuff or Your Life

We now have many more possessions in our homes than any society in history, and the rate of accumulation seems to be accelerating. We struggle to recycle, but we can't even manage the junk mail and packing materials, let alone our belongings. And yet we go on accumulating things as though our closets, basements and garages were bottomless. "Another trend that pointed to disaster," the archaeologists will say as they brush Styrofoam pellets off the sides of an ancient television. "Why didn't they see it coming?"

Indeed, you can anticipate various ergonomic flash points if you simply *promise yourself never to buy anything without first deciding where you will store it.* This is a crucial ergonomic issue; your peace of mind depends on it.

At the end of a long day you deserve to kick back and relax in your own living room. You shouldn't have to struggle to get up from the couch, and you shouldn't be expected to grapple with glare, noise and pollution.

Your back and neck shouldn't ache; your legs shouldn't go numb while you watch television.

The ergonomic challenge at home is to tune each room to the needs of your body. If you don't do it here, where will you do it?

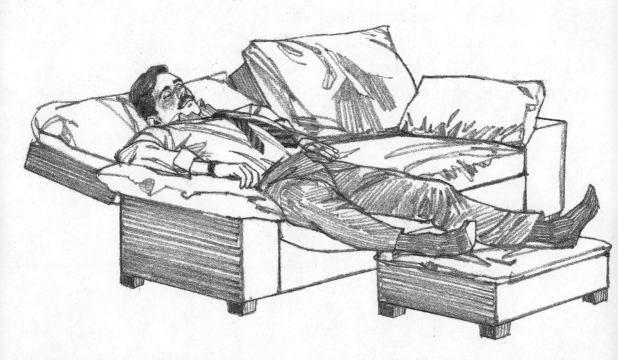

Living Room Storage: Things That Topple

Nothing undermines the living room as a place of peace and relaxation more thoroughly than mountains of toys, games, books, pens, newspapers, catalogs, tapes, CDs, records and videos piled on every flat surface. Annoying little piles of belongings will swell daily and topple without warning. Tapes slide under furniture, toys merge with books and periodicals, and precious floor space begins to disappear. Frantic cleanups begin an hour or so before guests arrive. Your meekest possessions have inherited your home, and you are at their mercy.

An ergonomic storage plan for the living room—a series of small steps—reclaims portions of the room you had abandoned to your possessions. Begin by eliminating junk. Your home cannot tolerate waste any better than your workplace. Be ruthless with your garbage; place a fairly large wastebasket next to each reading chair.

Everyone brings things into the living room and ideally each family member will agree to become responsible for his or her own garbage and storage. That simple formula can reduce tension more effectively than a month's worth of therapy. Start by making this simple agreement with everyone in your home, but remember, you will see little progress unless your living room storage has been tailored to the items you and your family actually use daily.

Magazine Storage

Slippery, thin magazines and catalogs are the most difficult to manage. Don't store them with books; they topple and slide relentlessly. Provide committed periodical readers with dedicated storage.

Each avid magazine reader should have an accompanying chair-side table with rear-sloping shelves to provide compact storage for magazines and catalogs. For more ambitious readers, use a library-style angled rack that keeps magazines clearly visible until you are ready to replace them with newer issues.

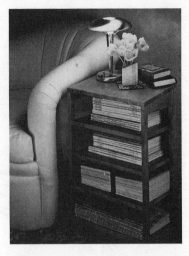

Most bookcase shelves are much too long. Lengthy rows of tilting books make book storage an unfriendly, difficult-to-manage process. Books get jammed randomly in place and forgotten. Eventually, your big books

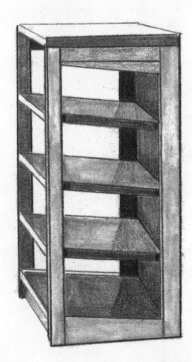

Levenger
420 Commerce Drive
Delray Beach, Florida 33445
(800) 544 0880

will put enough pressure on your little books to warp the bindings. The ergonomic solution, short cubicle-like shelves with dividers every twelve to fifteen inches, provides support

and rearranged easily. You can then add doors and glass windows and vary the shelf depths wherever necessary.

CDs and cassettes, with their tiny labels, become much easier

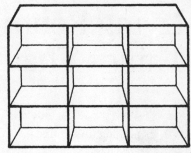

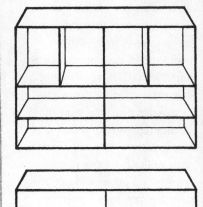

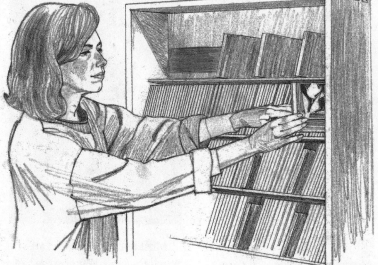

for your favorite volumes while making categorization much easier. Cubicle sizes can be tailored to fit various book heights. Make sure to provide long narrow spaces for atlases, oversize art books and game boxes. Adjustable dividers work well, though most people will stick with the initial settings for years.

Make sure your living room storage is movable, not just to a room down the hall but ultimately to another home. Heavy awkward furniture that's backbreaking to move is hopelessly unergonomic. You can easily fill a whole wall with modular pieces that once assembled look like a single unit. That kind of light, flexible system works better than a large, fixed bookcase. Small boxes geared to the item you wish to store can be stacked

to identify and handle when they are stored on rear-sloping shelves. Make sure good task lights illuminate each storage area. Without sufficient lighting the nasty little piles will return and begin to grow once again.

George Monroe Design
P.O. Box 584
Miranda, California 95553
(707) 943 3094

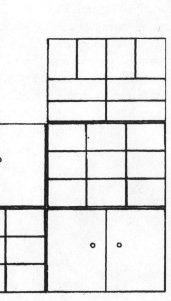

How to Talk

Do your dinner guests refuse to leave the dining room table? Do people jam themselves into your kitchen during parties while the rest of your home remains empty? Is everyone avoiding your living room?

Your problem isn't inertia; it's probably your couch.

The main purpose of the living room is to provide family and friends with a comfortable, inviting and cozy place to socialize. In our efforts to make the living room as comfortable as possible we emulate the most restful human environment, the bedroom. The living room as day bed is a stupifying place. We wallow in spongelike sofas and chairs which are arranged, theaterlike, in rows facing the television. We sit lined up like robots across the room, bumping thighs and elbows. Everything we touch collapses under us. In the name of comfort we sink so deeply into our chairs that the simple act of standing up becomes tricky. There are no firm surfaces in the living room as day bed, nothing to grasp. In deference to the television, the lights are dim. Conversation seems awkward, even rude— you could be interrupting an important show.

Sooner or later, those who are socially inclined retreat to the kitchen where they can look each other in the eye and talk.

The Antisocial Living Room

A couch that's too low

While an intimate couple may prefer a low divan to mull over the day or take a snooze, most people want eye contact during conversation. Attempting to look someone in the eye from a low couch strains the neck. Don't expect your guests to go through contortions to talk with each other.

Being forced into a half-reclining position also creates a feeling of vulnerability and misplaced intimacy. Your guests are more likely to end up in truly awkward positions. If the hips are too low and the knees are too high, clothes hike up. Don't permit your furniture to embarrass your guests.

A couch that's too soft

Furniture that's too low is generally too soft. The extra softness pitches strangers against each other, intensifying the problems of misplaced intimacy. Cushy furniture presents an even more challenging environment for elderly people and pregnant women. Even fixed-body activities like watching television become risky. Without lumbar support you cannot expect to hold any posture for long without risking injury.

A couch that's too deep

Low, soft and deep is the misguided formula for the ultimate in luxurious comfort. Dropping your guests into fetal-like positions near the floor simply aggravates all of the problems generated by soft and low cushions. Be ready to help people get back on their feet. Combining low, soft and deep seating in a television-dominated living room will guarantee a talkative crowd in your kitchen at every party.

Seating that's tight

"Built for five" promised the ad for your new L-shaped sofa, but it's seldom actually used by more than three. Yes, five family members can theoretically fit on the sofa, but what would they do then? A side-by-side seating position is needlessly crowded and awkward for conversation.

People don't like forced intimacy. In fact, your guests will go to great lengths to avoid touching each other. Strangers will choose to sit on the floor, a few feet away from each other, rather than brush knees and shoulders on your couch. The L-shaped sofa needs help from other furniture or it will become little more than an expensive conversation killer.

Seating that's too far apart

Your guests have a right to avoid forced intimacy. However, the horror of physical contact that seems to characterize our society can go too far. If people have to raise their voices to be heard, they are seated too far apart for conversation.

Conversation Enhancers

If you can't get rid of mushy, low furniture in your living room, add a few normal-height easy chairs to your conversation group. Well-constructed, high,

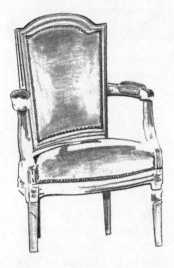

Your older friends as well as those who have a history of back problems will make a beeline for these chairs at every gathering. Plump individuals and pregnant women will follow. In

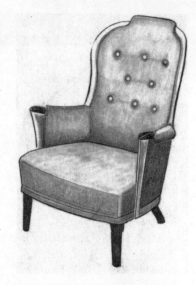

Interesting patterns emerge with movable chairs; watch how your guests arrange themselves. People prefer to sit at a slight angle to each other, not side-by-side or opposite one another. The round dining room table works well for conversation because of its friendly shape. Ovals, horseshoes and gently rounded furniture configurations promote conversation while angular, square or rectangular shapes discourage it.

straight-backed chairs with firm padding and lumbar support will encourage your guests to relax and talk with each other. An ottoman to rest the feet makes the chair even more inviting.

fact, all of your guests will appreciate sensible straight-backed chairs. Add soft, large pillows to the low furniture you insist on keeping. If you want your guests to talk, prop them up so they can see each other.

How to Read

If you like to read, you probably read everywhere —in bed, over breakfast, in the bathroom, on the couch, in a bookstore, on an airplane. Perhaps you make do with inadequate ambient illumination or with a dim light from a purely decorative table lamp.

Most likely, you're so absorbed in your reading that you pay little attention to the awkward postures you assume. You might slump for hours in a sagging, overstuffed couch, sprawl across a bed, or scan a book while pedaling an exercise machine. Reading, as you know, is one of life's great pleasures— there should be no penalty for enjoying it. Your eyes shouldn't burn the next morning. Your neck and back shouldn't stiffen every time you open a book.

You owe it to yourself to create a comfortable and ergo-nomic reading habitat. While you're at it, create ergonomic reading habitats for your children too. Spontaneous reading will follow.

We have already seen how bad ergonomics can cause needless strife in a family. Somehow the innocent things everyone takes for granted— mail, shoes, toys, sports equipment, pillows, closets—seem to cause the most trouble. In fact, even the simple act of reading a book can ruin a quiet evening at home if a few people try to read in the same room.

Is your couch flanked by intense reading lamps? When two people try reading together in this familiar setting with difficult-to-adjust lamps set up at opposite ends of a couch, at least one of them will be looking sideways into a naked light bulb. L-shaped couches bring

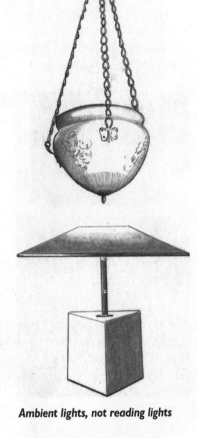

Ambient lights, not reading lights

the tormenting light closer to front and center where it can blast you right in the face. In order to illuminate a few square inches of paper, people end up flooding half a room with unshaded light at intensities usually reserved for police interrogation cells. Decorator magazines are overflowing with poorly lighted couches on which families presumably struggle nightly as they slowly go blind.

If you acquire just one ergonomic criterion from this book, remember this: decorative lamps and ceiling lights provide ambient light, good for locating large objects like children. They are hopeless for reading.

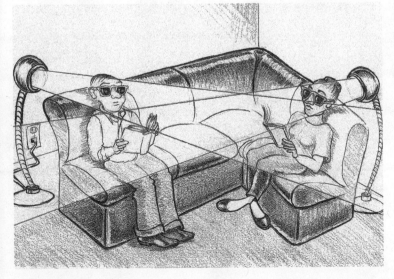

Your Personal Chair

A personal ergonomic chair, more than any other object, defines your sense of well-being. Settling into it becomes a sensual experience, an unmistakable pleasure that you will look forward to all day. In fact, without

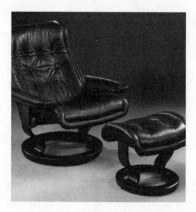

an ergonomic chair to relax in you will never feel as though you actually belong in your own home. Choose your chair carefully; it's your ergonomic sanctuary from the insults of the day.

You will want to do many things in your chair so be sure it's adjustable and fitted to your needs. Keep models that are stingy, underpadded torture racks, overstuffed monsters and angular disasters out of your home.

Your Own Reading Light

Each reader in your family has the right to a narrow-beam adjustable reading light with a metal head that stays cool to the touch. In a dimly lighted room each lamp creates a pool of light just wide enough to illuminate a large book. When a reader can share a couch with a music lover who prefers soft lighting, you have the makings of a truly civilized evening.

A Good Chair Should . . .

Embrace you
supporting your whole body from head to foot

Swivel
and remain comfortable while you recline

Elevate
your head sufficiently while reclining to read or watch television

Include
a separate, padded footstool. Avoid the one-piece joined chaise and footrest that supports your feet when you recline only to leave them dangling when you sit up to read.

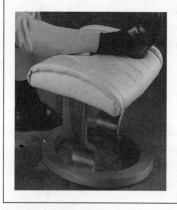

Ekornes Inc.
500 Memorial Drive
Somerset, New Jersey 08873
(800) 356 7637

To make sure the light won't disturb others, choose a lamp with a small, well-shaded, flexible head and bring the head to within a few feet of your book when you read. A dimmer gives you added flexibility but isn't essential. Flexible lamps with shaded heads (often with twelve-volt tungsten bulbs) are available in floor and table models.

Beware of flimsy task lights with difficult-to-adjust heads. Avoid any lamp that fights back when you aim it. Be sure the beam of light is narrow rather than wide-angled.

Before you buy a lamp, try it while seated in a reading chair. The illuminated head should stay exactly where you put it without resisting or springing

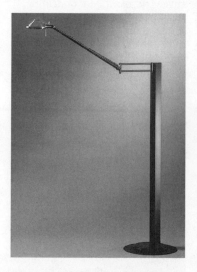

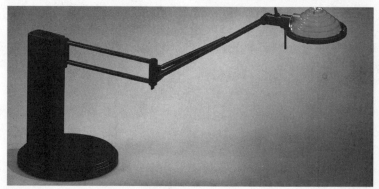

back to a preset position. Once the lamp is in your reading position, the bulb itself should be invisible from any other chair in the room. Expect to move the lamp head frequently; look for high-quality hardware and a well-shielded bulb, especially on halogen lamps, which get very hot.

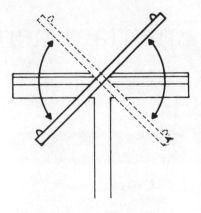

Luxo Lamp Company
36 Midland Avenue
Port Chester, New York 10573
(914) 937 4433

Things That Tilt

You read best when your material is on the same plane as your eyes; reading only becomes a chore when you must bend your neck forward. We all understand the importance of taking a break from desk work in the office, but it seems redundant to take a break from relaxing with a good book at home. Nevertheless, when you settle down in an easy chair with a good book for a few hours, your neck and shoulders are under constant assault.

Think of an ergonomic read-ing chair as an essential tool that may require a bit of fine tuning. When you're seated, your neck and back will be properly supported for hours of nearly motionless activity. Reading, however, isn't quite motionless. The innocent act of lifting up a book and holding it in place at the right angle can undermine the best chair. Hours go by while your hands, arms, neck and shoulders are locked in tension to accommo-date a tiny inanimate object—a classic ergonomic error.

Happily, a number of simple

To spare your arms, support your book with a reading pillow (below); a reading table holds your book at the proper angle (right).

reading tools are now available to keep your book from tortur-ing your body.

The ergonomic solution, plac-ing the book on an adjustable platform, spares your neck and shoulders. Adjustable reading tools range from small portable units that fit in your lap or can be set up on a desktop, to roll-around units that tuck in below your chest while you're seated. The larger units have an addi-tional shelf space for drinks, note pads or reading glasses. What they all have in common is the ability to support your book at the right angle, so your body isn't held in a tense posi-tion for hours at a time.

More elaborate reading tables combine tilted reading surfaces with storage for books and refer-ence materials. Here, too, you should be able to rest your arms, as well as your neck and shoul-ders, while you read.

Levenger
420 Commerce Drive
Delray Beach, Florida 33445
(800) 544 0880

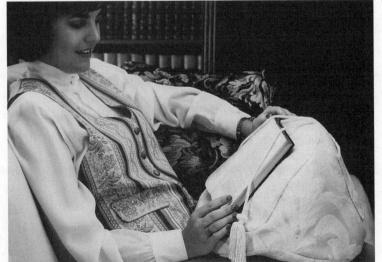

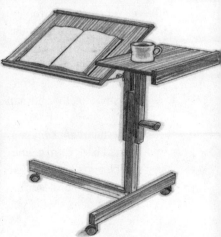

The Greedy Entertainment Center

The entertainment center, consisting of a television and audio system, has replaced the hearth at the center of the American home. This is where we do our most serious relaxing. But just as the home computer has begun to take over the bedroom, the entertainment center has begun a relentless assault on the living room. Before you set up the rear-projection television and the trunk-size speakers, think carefully about how you want to spend your time at home. The choices you make will determine what goes on in your living room.

You need open space for children to play, or they won't. If you give children space directly in front of a twenty-seven-inch television, they will watch television instead of reading, playing, talking or exercising. You need space in your living room to read, or you won't. And you need a way for people to talk with each other, or they won't. The choice comes down to this: are you going to dedicate the most important room in your home to mountains of electronic equipment or to other human beings?

Your entertainment center can be moved back from center stage; in fact, parts of it can disappear altogether. The assumption that we humans should get out of the way of our own enter-

The Spec Trap

Technological perfection

Modern audio/visual components are built to degrees of perfection that are no longer detectable by human beings. You might be able to tell the difference between distortion levels of 1% and 10%, but no human being can detect the difference between .009% and .002%, an "improvement" quoted to sell stereo equipment.[1] You're expected to bury yourself in charts of technical specifications (affectionately known as "specs"), comparing long lists of virtually identical numbers. This techno-worship that rules the world of consumer electronics, is meant to convince you that the equipment itself is beautiful enough to be on view in your home. We are expected to appreciate the blinking lights and swinging meters and stare at menu-laden LED screens while we listen to music.

The real test

Resist the temptation to select equipment based on specifications that have no bearing on the way you entertain yourself. Filling your living room with technically perfect machines will do nothing for your body. The only test to discover the differences between these products is ergonomic. But that may be the last thing the manufacturer wants you to think about.

tainment center is a carryover from the uncompromising world of the audiophile, where electronic behemoths are set up in the center of a room, and rope-thick cables snake shamelessly across the rug. Racks of glowing light-emitting diodes (LEDs), swinging meters, bar graphs and purple-yellow radio tubes remain in full view where they can be openly worshipped. And of course money is no object.

The audiophile cheerfully pulls apart his home to achieve sonic perfection and heaven help the spouse who objects. Now you are expected to do the same thing by the makers of the home theater. In a commercial theater, you aren't permitted to do anything but watch the movie. This is the atmosphere you're being asked to create in your living room.

If you crave the feeling of being enveloped in gigantic video images accompanied by eight-speaker surround sound, dedicate a separate room to your equipment. Go there and be enveloped. But don't try to turn your living room into a theater, lest it actually become one.

1. Just a few years ago such differences were undetectable by laboratory instruments.

Things That Go Boom

As new semiconductor chips are developed and more features added, the home entertainment system is becoming a Christmas tree of blinking lights and swinging meters. But what we see on our space-age audiovisual control center is seldom what we get. Our favorite program somehow doesn't get recorded on time, the system switches on by itself—to the wrong station—and the remote control clatters to the floor every time we reach for it. Boom boom goes the self-powered woofer, and shortly after that the neighbors begin pounding on the walls. Thanks to hopeless ergonomics, even home entertainment becomes a stressful routine.

It's an expensive lesson. The great features that held such promise in the store are seldom used. We skip the lengthy instruction manual, managing only to turn the machine on, select a program and set the volume. The *user interface* (the controls that human beings must learn in order to operate the machine) is just too difficult.

Put ergonomics first when buying a music system, television, VCR or any other component. The user interface has two parts: the remote control and the main unit. Generally, the remote duplicates the controls on the main unit. You need the following essential ergonomic

features to enjoy an entertainment system.

Simplicity

Eliminate all unnecessary steps. You shouldn't have to press *on* first, and then *radio*. Pressing *radio* should turn on that component. Similarly, you shouldn't have to turn off one component (for example, the CD control) to turn on a radio or tape recorder. Pressing a new source should shut off the old source while starting the new one. While you don't need a separate *on* button, you will require a common *off* button.

Layering

The main unit should work on a layering principle in which only the basic controls needed to start the system (radio, tape, CD, etc.) are always visible. Additional controls become visible when you need them. For example, if you press *tape*, you should then see only icons for *play, fast forward, rewind*

and *record* on the display of the main unit.

Standardized Icons

These help make the controls easy to find and operate, especially when the lights are low.

Foolproof Controls

Your system should anticipate common mistakes and ensure that it cannot be accidentally defeated. Pressing the *record* button during a radio show, for example, should begin the recording process, not shut off the radio and turn on the tape recorder.

Visible and Handy Controls

Controls should be easy to use by normal adult-size hands. Beware of clustered buttons, sliders or knobs that provide poor tactile feedback. If you must study banks of tiny controls with a flashlight and magnifying glass, you don't have an ergonomic user interface.

Inconspicuous Components

The user interface shouldn't be seen or heard when you're listening to music. At a live performance you watch the performer, not the amplification equipment. The less you have to consult your user interface, the more ergonomic it becomes. Your home entertainment components should look like furniture, not cockpit controls.

Shopping for an Audio System

When shopping for an audio system, good sound is a given; the important questions are purely ergonomic. Before you buy, tear yourself away from the "spec" sheets and glossy photos and consider how you actually operate the equipment. If the unit seems too complex in a showroom, you will probably never memorize or use all of its functions.

Start by evaluating the remote control, the most essen-

Weighted to fit in your hand, this remote permits your fingers to curl naturally onto the rubberized controls.

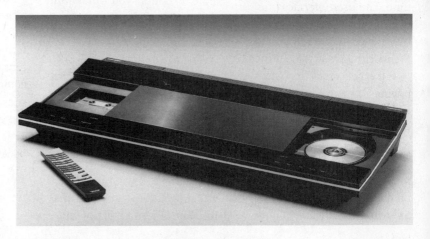

tial ergonomic audio component and the most frequently handled part of the user interface. Like any hand tool it must be balanced, or you will drop it. It should also be weighted to fit your grip and thin enough to be held comfortably in one hand. Make sure it has tactile features so you can find various functions in the dark. Rubberized buttons are helpful, as are varied shapes like up- and down-facing triangles for increasing and decreasing volume. Ideally, its body should reflect light; white or metallic surfaces work well. A black remote might match your stereo, but it will be difficult to locate in a dimly lit room. Beware of button-studded, flat plastic remotes. Your fingers should fall naturally on the most often-used controls: on-off, volume and source

The ergonomic audio system: one cabinet, one power cord, no buttons

(radio, tape, CD and so on). A remote with standard icons to match those on the main unit makes the operation easier. Controls for complex systems, say, multiroom audio plus video, should be layered. The most *often* used—not the easiest—controls should be in clear view, and the most infrequently used—not the most difficult—ones should be concealed beneath a subpanel.

What do you actually need in a remote? Everything beyond on-off capabilities, volume, mute and program selection is seldom used. Obscure controls don't have to be at your fingertips every moment. Thus, often-used features like *on* and *radio* require large dedicated buttons while each of the less frequently used features (like the edit

Bang & Olufsen
1150 Feehanville Drive
Mount Prospect, Illinois 60056
(800) 323 0378

control) can be assigned a single button and moved to a hidden subpanel. This is precisely the solution Bang & Olufsen devised for their home entertainment systems. By setting up

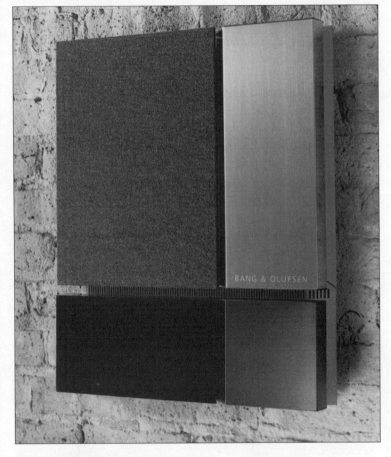

The speaker as art instead of obelisk

a system of ergonomic priorities, they managed to make multiroom equipment, which is usually far more complex than an ordinary audiovisual system, much easier to use. Virtually any command can be executed with large, dedicated, color-coded, labeled buttons. On more complex models, infrequently used buttons are hidden beneath a subpanel.

Resist audio snobbery when selecting components. Models that bristle with knobs, dials and sliders generally sound identical

to "basic" units; the complex systems will simply be much more difficult to operate. Racks of blinking components have no legitimate claim on your habitat. Most visible controls, including

tiny meters and banks of LEDs, are unreadable from more than a few feet away. Use them when you need them, for example, during a recording session, and tuck them away when you don't. In fact, the only objects you must see from your listening position are your speakers, which ideally can be built into the walls and even disguised as art or wallpaper.

Three-piece systems with

separate subwoofers (for low frequencies) provide an elegant solution for those who do not wish to remodel. The large subwoofer boxes, which work perfectly well when concealed under furniture, significantly reduce the size of the visible speaker, a further ergonomic advantage. You see only a pair of shoe box–size satellite speakers, which produce the high frequencies.

Whenever you remodel, string speaker wire through the exposed walls from room to room, whether you need it immediately or not. To prevent an audible hum from entering your system, keep speaker wires at least a foot away from household electrical wires.

Consolidate your equipment as much as possible in a single cabinet. A separate power supply and cabinet for a tuner, CD, cassette and amplifier will only complicate your habitat and raise the electric bill.

In time, all audio components end up covered with a carpet of dust. Rather than passively accepting this evolution, set up all your wiring so that each component can be moved easily and vacuumed.

How to Watch Television

Whether or not your television is integrated into a home entertainment system, its ergonomic consequences must be considered separately. Television is an addictive device that has a way of putting an end to social interaction. We all know the dangers of overindulgence: bored, overweight children and strangely passive and depressed adults.

Television, however, is not evil incarnate, merely another demanding machine that needs to be pushed back from the center of your habitat. Adults and especially children should have to make a conscious decision to watch a show.

Any activity that freezes your

Television has replaced the hearth at the center of the American home.

body into a single posture for hours on end is potentially dangerous. This is not an argument against television itself; air travel and reading are equally hard on the body. With air travel, however, we deal with the hazards of inactivity; we will exercise occasionally, both on and off the airplane, to restore circulation and muscle tone. But the fact that television locks your body in place as surely as a dentist's chair simply isn't widely recognized. You shouldn't have to pay a physical and mental penalty for a few hours of entertainment. Good ergonomics will make television much easier on your mind and body.

Hide the television when it's not in use; it shouldn't be permitted to dominate a room. The ideal ergonomic solution is to dedicate a room to it. If you can't arrange a completely separate space, set up the television in a cabinet with doors that can be closed. To increase the flexibility of your home, isolate the television from other living room activities. Set it up on a rolling TV cart that can be pushed into a corner of the room and covered with a cloth. At all costs avoid the classic ergonomic error: letting your television drone on in the background while you attempt to do other things.

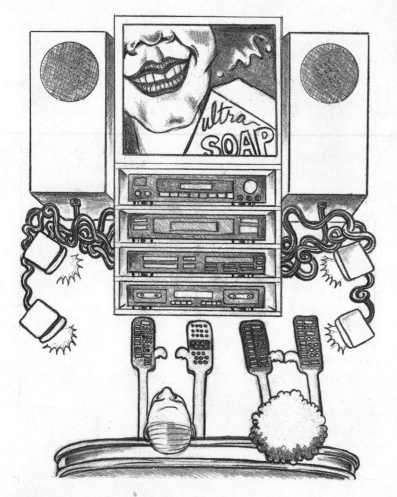

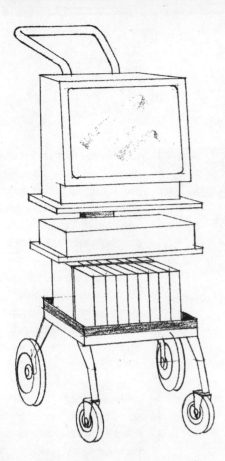

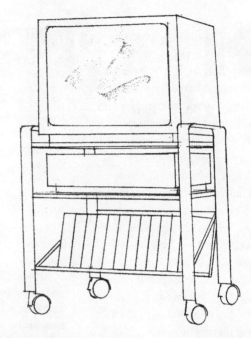

Never watch television while tilting your face upward. Sprawling on the floor in front of a television, a favorite position of small children, means maintaining an upward tilt in your neck for hours, which can cause cervical pain. Half lying or half sitting on a sagging couch affects adults similarly.

Sit, don't slump, in a chair or couch with good lumbar and neck support. Don't hesitate to use pillows to help create lumbar support in a deep couch. Elevate your legs. Using a recliner or ottoman to support your legs relieves pressure on your neck and lower back while improving blood circulation. Take frequent breaks during which you can walk and stretch your limbs.

Television screens emit the same low-frequency electromagnetic waves that worry computer users (see p. 166). Fortunately, the radiation levels virtually disappear about three feet from the screen, another reason for keeping your children away from the set.

If you dine in front of the television, place your food on a table that's high enough so you don't have to bend down while eating. Staring up at the television while bending down to eat is a sure recipe for back pain. Sit upright in a chair with good lumbar back support.

To control glare, eliminate light sources that are reflected in your screen and brightly lighted areas behind the television.

Control your quality time (and zoom through commercials) with a VCR. Television prime time seems to coincide with prime time at home—dinnertime, bedtime for children, visits with friends. Recording your favorite programs permits you to watch them when they don't interfere with your social and educational activities.

Selecting a VCR

Most people never learn to operate a VCR. The instruction booklet is too long, the remote control too complex and the unit itself too puzzling to use beyond the most basic level. Although tens of millions of VCRs have been sold, it is an acknowledged ergonomic failure.

Nevertheless, manufacturers keep adding new features, thus making the user interface even more complicated. A machine that is used daily should be as unambiguous and straightforward to use as an alarm clock. Keep this in mind when you shop for a new unit. Like digital watches, cameras and CD players, the technical capabilities of most VCRs are roughly equal. You pay extra for poor ergonomics.

Apart from handling the cassette, most VCR operations are performed with the remote control. VCR ergonomics thus focuses on the design of this essential tool.

Be sure your remote operates on standard infrared frequencies so you can replace it easily if it fails. "Universal" remotes, designed to operate many different units, often make a difficult VCR even harder to use. Try the remote before purchasing it and ask yourself whether or not it actually makes common operations easier. Simply adding more controls will complicate any machine. Sadly, you're better off with separate ergonomic remotes than a complex universal model.

Remotes that are keyed to newspaper codes make time programming easier, an ergonomic plus. Make sure, however, that the essential daily controls haven't become more difficult.

Test the remote with your eyes closed. Look for the same tactile features you required on audio remotes (see p. 78). The essential controls you will use daily, like *play, pause* and *rewind*, should be immediately obvious. Again, the remote should be balanced to fit in your hand like a fine knife or hammer. Avoid flat plastic rectangles with banks of identical buttons.

Cordless Headphones

Despite their great sound quality, headphones are seldom used for serious listening. Corded headphones force you to sit within a few feet of the music source, which is poor ergonomics. Even when extended, the cord (and thus the headphone itself) becomes inconvenient.

Now, thanks to full-range cordless headphones, which are sonically far superior to in-the-ear "bud" headphones used with portables, you can listen to Coltrane full volume at midnight without having to apologize to the neighbors.

A small infrared or FM trans-mitter plugs into the earphone jack on your music source or television. The battery-powered headphones contain a tiny receiver that picks up high-fidelity sound anywhere in a large living room. Unlike corded units, the volume is controlled from the headphones themselves. This adds the basic remote-control features of portable tape and CD players to your home, an important ergonomic advantage. It also eliminates complex television and audio remotes which are unnecessary for listening or viewing a single source. When you're finished listening, you simply turn off the headphones.

Cordless headphones bring high-quality personal music to the bedroom (see p. 97) as well as the living room.

 Koss Corporation
4129 North Port Washington Avenue
Milwaukee, Wisconsin 53212
(800) USA KOSS

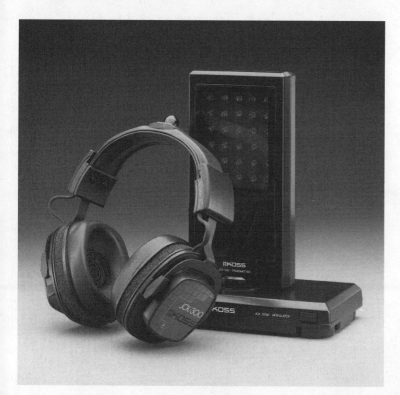

Wiring and Cables

Simply cramming a tangled mass of wires and cables behind the entertainment system may seem like a small price to pay for your hard-won hours of relaxation. It is, in fact, a classic ergonomic error.

No matter how many outlets you have, lamp cords most likely already frame part of your living room. Each new piece of audiovisual equipment unavoidably introduces new wires and cables. Stuffed out of sight, they join lamp cords and speaker wires behind the living room furniture to form a twisted mass known as *spaghetti*. The moment you abandon a space to wiring you lose control of the wiring.

Furthermore, in a few weeks those unimportant-looking few inches behind the entertainment center will be filled with dust balls and debris. Routine cleaning is abandoned because it means loosening crucial connections. Vacuum the living room as much as you like; allergy sufferers will still feel the presence of hidden dust the moment they enter the room. And you will too, sooner or later.

To accept spaghetti in your living room is to surrender to chaos. Since it isn't possible to eliminate all the wires, you must manage them more effectively. The industrial solution— flexible plastic tubes called *wire guides*, works as well in the home as it does in the factory. A half dozen or more sets of wires fit through each flexible tube, emerging through strategic slits at an outlet or nearby component. Complex systems may

need more than one tube. Wire guides are easy to clean with a vacuum or by hand. When the time comes, sets of wires can be easily extracted or exchanged. One thick tube replaces a mass of tangled wires.

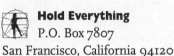 **Hold Everything**
P.O. Box 7807
San Francisco, California 94120
(800) 421 2264

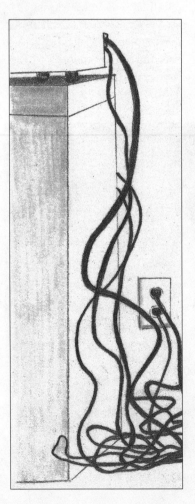 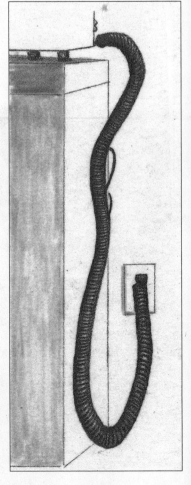

84

5. How to Sleep

One thing is certain in America: the quality and quantity of sleep obtained are substantially less than the quality and quantity that are needed. Over the past century, we have reduced our average nightly total sleep time by more than 20 percent. . . . A substantial number of people—perhaps the majority—are functionally handicapped by sleep deprivation on any given day.[1] ❦ In sleep our brilliance, wit and accomplishments are denied expression. We can never see ourselves asleep. It is unthinkable that the sprawling, vegetating, perhaps snoring sleeper is the real thing. Thus it is only human to regard sleep as a strange interruption of the waking state in which we are "ourselves." ❦ But it is just as reasonable to regard wakefulness as an interruption of the sleeping state. Fetal life is a sleeping life and it is amazing that the fetus continues its sleep even during labor unless aroused by threatened asphyxia.[2]

1. DR. WILLIAM DEMENT, "Wake Up America: A National Sleep Alert," *Stanford Observer,* January-February, 1993.

2. *The Anatomy of Sleep,* Roche Laboratories, Division of Hoffmann-LaRoche Inc., Nutley, New Jersey, 1966.

The Bedroom Habitat

The bedroom is an ergonomic disaster zone, a place where nightly accidents occur, a venue for silent punishment. If we realized the dangers that await us after dark, we would march into the bedroom with a fire ax. Instead, we tiptoe around it with interior decorating magazines, hanging pictures, plumping pillows and casting little throw rugs around at interesting angles. The result is a lovely stage set called *the decorator's dream* into which we drop our exhausted bodies every evening, expecting relief.

When the lights go down, the set closes in on us. We grapple with sleep on taut, unforgiving mattresses mounted in gargantuan frames. We clean fastidiously around untouched mountains of debris. We develop weird allergies, flulike symptoms or insomnia. We wrestle half-consciously with piles of unruly blankets and giant, overstuffed pillows. We crowd in magazines, plants, trophies, souvenirs, cosmetics, pets, food and toys. And we long for the servants and full-time housewives who once kept it all in order. We charge up little appliances on the night table; we wrap ourselves in electric blan-

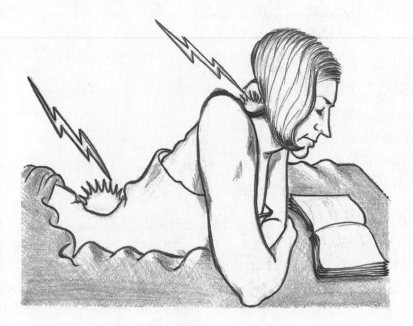

The Four Bedroom Zones

1. The inner zone
Bed frame:
light and movable
Mattress:
hard beds stay hard
Covered comforter:
bed making in thirty seconds
Pillows:
soft and full body support
Headboard:
adjustable back support

2. The reachable zone
Reading light:
narrow beam and adjustable
Reading table:
movable and adjustable
Alarm clock:
tactile controls
Entertainment system:
remote and cordless

3. The storage zone
Clothes valet:
men, women and children
Personal hamper:
good for your clothes and
your relationship
Wardrobe:
it's 6:00 A.M., do you know
where your clothes are?

4. The invisible zone
Air quality:
dust and mite control
Sound:
good noise, bad noise and
privacy

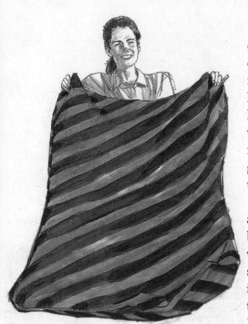

kets and crank up the current. Our heads twisted at precarious angles, we fumble with books and newspapers, squinting at the tiny print. We stare straight ahead through the darkness, hour after hour, into giant, luminous television screens.

We seem to be spending enough time in bed—why then do we run out of energy every day; why are we tired all the time? Sleep deprivation could be the most serious unacknowledged health problem in the country today.

Our bedrooms are traditional and outmoded. For centuries, the bedroom has remained an overdecorated nighttime storage space for the body, a place where style rules. We have lavished attention on our furniture and wall hangings, our rugs and decorative pillows, but we have granted our sleeping bodies no legitimate rights of their own. So we suffer, even when doing nothing. Our Victorian ancestors would have approved.

From the bed to the outside walls, the ergonomic bedroom meets the needs of the human body. You may have to be ruthless with your existing bedroom to achieve this goal, but you have a lot to gain.

You probably spend as much time in your bedroom as you do at work. In fact, your sleeping environment influences your mood throughout the day.

Just because your body is passive and at the mercy of the immediate environment doesn't mean you should ignore its needs. Once again, your ergonomic rights begin at the walls of the room.

Divide the bedroom habitat into four zones. The innermost one contains your bed and bedding; the second, everything you must be able to reach while in bed: a night table, lamp, clock radio, books and storage for personal items like medication. The third zone contains your dressers and closets, and the fourth, at the windows and walls of your room, is the invisible zone of air, climate and sound.

Using the ergonomic guidelines that follow, look closely first at the innermost zone: the bed and mattress you now own. We hesitate to keep a car for ten, fifteen or twenty years; why expect more from a mattress? Most of us sleep on the same mattress far too long.

Bedroom Health Risks and Solutions

Backache	Level, resilient bed suited to your body type and high enough to get out of easily
Stiff neck	Soft, malleable double pillow set; adjustable backrest for reading and watching television; adjustable bed lamp; tilting book tray or nightstand; adjustable wall-mounted TV with remote control
Poor circulation	Level, resilient, soft bed suited to your body type; light bedding that doesn't restrict movement
Allergies (*sneezing, ichy eyes/skin, fatigue, irritability*)	Easy-to-clean bed and bedroom; good ventilation; hypoallergenic materials
No privacy	Soundproofing; white noise machine; cordless headphones
Sleeping problems	All of the above

Your Sleep Profile

The more you resemble an hourglass, the more demanding you will be of your mattress. Conversely, the more you resemble a sweet potato, the less demanding you will be of your bed. Slender people (especially thin men with wide shoulders), pregnant women and the elderly require *soft, resilient,* high-quality mattresses. Beware of puritanical mattress advertising: any of the "superfirm" or harder varieties that promise "natural" sleep postures will bring nights of unrelenting torture.

Generally, the thinner you are, the more you will appreciate a softer mattress. Pay close attention to the protruding parts of your body when testing a mattress. Unsupported male shoulders will easily twist the spine on an unforgiving mattress. A woman's body generally requires additional cushioning, particularly if she has recently given birth. If your pelvic bones have been forced far apart during childbirth, a pillow held between or under your thighs will reduce the discomfort of sleeping on a hard mattress.

Your Habitual Sleeping Position

Anything that restricts your activity in bed detracts from the quality of your sleep. We change position during sleep at least ten times every night when we are well, more than one hundred times when we are sick, worried or attempting to sleep on a hard or sagging bed. A good mattress will permit you to sleep through this necessary movement.

An ergonomic mattress must be *soft* enough to give way to the protruding parts of your body, *resilient* enough to support the concave parts while keeping the spine straight and *firm* enough for you to roll over easily.

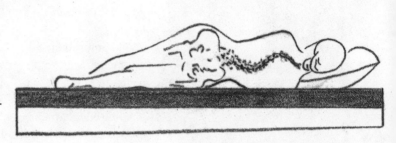

Too hard

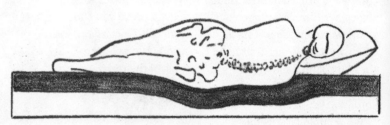

Too soft

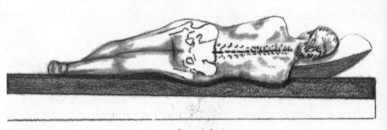

Just right

A Bed for Your Body

The American bed seeks to emulate the grand beds of European aristocracy, a useful role model if you have servants and plan to stay where you are forever. If you don't, the sheer bulk and weight of an oversize frame and mattress can make the bed a permanent fixture in your home long after its useful life has ended. Once your mattress sags even a little, it's worn out, and it will never again give you a good night's sleep. You must get rid of it.

Are extra-firm beds somehow better designed and worth a premium price? You may not be completely satisfied with your posture (few of us are), but the bed is not the place for radical corrective measures. Suffering through the night on a rock-hard mattress won't straighten your back or "align" your spine, but it definitely will keep you tossing and turning for hours.

There is no law that says you cannot have a small, light bed. Although stand-alone futons are usually too firm, simply adding a corrugated sheet of foam rubber known as an *egg-crate topper* (see p. 92) generally provides resilience, an essential ergonomic feature that allows a bed to shape itself to the human body (more on resilience later). A frame with flexible slats permits you to customize a bed without the bulk and weight of standard innerspring models.

Above all else, a mattress must not twist the spine. Since the spine and neck must remain straight while the hips and shoulders are cushioned, the best mattress will shape itself to the contour of your body. Think first about the most important ergonomic relationship for sleepers, the one between the interior of a mattress and your spine. Get it right and you will change your life. Ignore it and you will suffer daily.

Beds: Basic Ergonomics

Bed must be level

Don't try to adapt to a sway-backed bed. Correct minor sagging with a bed board. Use braced 3/4-inch plywood or a material of equivalent strength. If your bed sags badly, look for a new one.

Hard and soft

The mattress itself must *give* to accommodate protruding parts of your body like the shoulders and hips.

Support

The mattress must support the convex parts of your body like the waist and knees.

Resiliency

The mattress must be resilient enough to follow the natural curves of your body. Flexibility, not rigidity, will keep your spine straight.

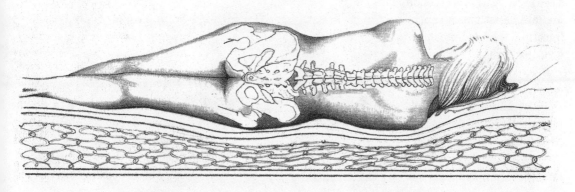

How to Test a Mattress

Choosing a mattress on the first bounce is like buying a car without driving it. The ergonomic question to ask in the bedroom is not whether or not you can manage to fall asleep but what *quality* of sleep you will experience. Deep sleep thoroughly rests your body, leaving it invigorated upon waking. Light, restless sleep leaves you fatigued and irritable, a feeling that has a way of lingering all through the following day. Tests have shown that an ergonomic mattress will provide about 25 percent more deep sleep than a standard mattress.

Unless you're ready to stay put all night, avoid hammocks and camp beds, which force your body into a fixed position. Never confuse a soft mattress with a sagging one. A good soft mattress or water bed molds itself to the contours of your body and provides from 10 to 25 percent more deep sleep each night. This adds up to weeks, even months, of additional deep sleep every year. Few ergonomic improvements have as much impact on your daily health as a good mattress.

A decent mattress evaluation requires getting very relaxed and if possible actually simulating real sleep. In a reasonably peaceful atmosphere you can do this in a few minutes. Keep in mind, however, that most mat-

Test a Mattress by:

Touching it
Is it smooth and soft when touched lightly? Does it give under light pressure?

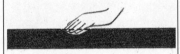

Lying down on it
Using a pillow—you won't feel comfortable on any bed without one—assume your usual sleeping position. Does the mattress allow your hips and shoulders to sink in while gently supporting your waist and legs? Does your spine feel comfortable?

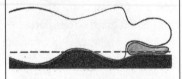

Sitting up on it
Do you bottom out? The mattress will punish you if your body can feel the frame or bed board.

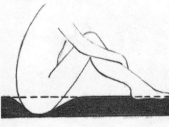

SOURCE: Möbelinstitutet, Stockholm, Sweden

tress shops, whether by accident or design, do not provide the ideal atmosphere to evaluate a bed. You cannot expect to relax properly while a salesperson leans over you in a brightly lighted, cavernous showroom, order pad in hand. Pressured and slightly embarrassed, you will rush when you should rest.

A flop-and-wiggle mattress evaluation—two minutes each on the back and stomach—will usually convince you that the brochure is right about the deluxe model. Then comes the battle to "break in" an unfriendly mattress, fought in your own bedroom soon afterward. Night after night, your restless body presses down hard, while unforgiving springs fight back. The loser will develop accommodating new curves.

Make a conscious effort to slow down when you test a bed. Turn on your side, the position most people use when sleeping. The belly is the second most common position, the back a distant third. Since sleep is far from static—you will probably move a couple of times each hour—plan on rolling around.

Happily, the fourteen most common positions (see p. 91) have been identified and provide a convenient basis for testing the ergonomic quality of any mattress. You're not likely to find them posted in your mattress showroom so bring this book to the store, send the salesperson out for coffee and try them all.

While sleeping on your side, you probably raise your knees, concentrating the weight of the thighs and midsection in one place. This position increases pressure by 25 percent (over a stretched-out position) on the portion of the mattress around your hips. If you are part of the 70 percent of the public who prefers sleeping this way, be certain to choose a mattress with good molding qualities. A softer-than-normal mattress will accept increased pressure at the hips while keeping you comfortable. If you feel a squeezing or numbing sensation at your elbows, shoulders, hips and knees, the mattress is too hard.

When you sleep on your side, the thinner parts of your body at the waist and legs create exaggerated curves. A soft mattress must also be resilient, able to mold itself to the changing shapes of your body that require support.

Mattress Toppers

Choosing an overly firm mattress, one of the most common ergonomic mistakes in the bedroom, can ruin your health. A comfortable mattress must permit you to move during sleep *while it supports your body*. You get the movement on a hard mattress without the support. Sleeping becomes a gymnastic effort: you will pitch back and forth all night long trying to get comfortable.

Researchers have found that sleepers will turn ten times more often on a hard mattress

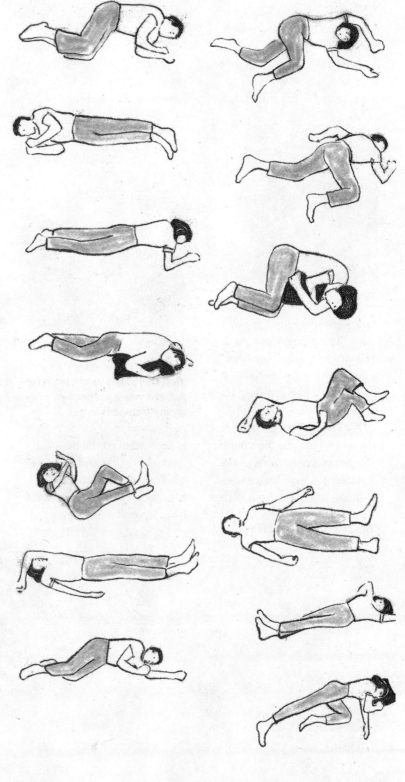

The fourteen most common sleeping positions

Source: Wennergren Institute, Stockholm, Sweden

than on a soft one. With your circulation cut off and your back twisted out of shape, the whole process of sleeping is degraded. But don't blame yourself for waking up feeling stiff and

of changing beds. It's a quick fix for sleepless nights.

The soft peaked foam tops give way where needed and provide support elsewhere; look for resiliency in a topper. The

with the little foam cones pointed up. With this ergonomic addition, a hard, unforgiving bed suddenly seems to contour itself to your body. You will feel the difference immediately.

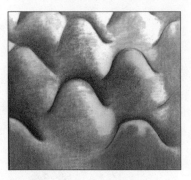

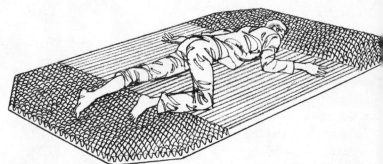

irritable, with nagging aches and pains that refuse to go away. Blame your mattress. You simply cannot "break in" a superfirm mattress the way you would a pair of shoes. Hard beds stay hard.

A convoluted foam mattress topper can provide the missing support you need to stay comfortable on a hard mattress—without the expense and bother

This bed includes a topper.

Most thin foam sheets used in toppers last only a year or two. High-quality foam lasts longer.

spaces between the peaks improve airflow and regulate your body temperature while you sleep. Select a topper made from hypoallergenic material and place it on your mattress

Self Care Catalog
5850 Shellmound Street
Emeryville, California 94662
(800) 345 3371

Duxiana
305 East 63rd Street
New York, New York 10021
(212) 752 3897

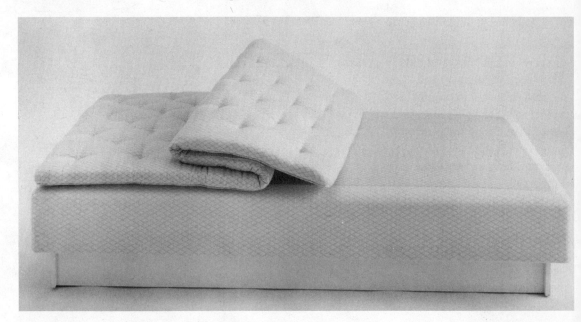

Choosing the Right Pillow

The next time you reach for an aspirin with your morning coffee, consider whether or not your neck has been bent out of shape for the past eight hours. You cannot achieve peace of mind if you sleep on the wrong pillow.

Your head is a heavy object and you must rest it on something when you sleep. But the real job of a pillow is to support the neck as well as the head. Other parts of your body may also require cushioning. Specialized pillows for the knees and whole body may add to your comfort at night. Try them all.

Think first about your head and neck. Not even the most ergonomically correct mattress can be expected to properly support the bony parts of your body without a pillow or two. The wrong pillow forces your neck into an awkward position for hours on end. With a pillow that's too low, your upper body begins to resemble a kind of tortured suspension bridge, touching the mattress at the center of the skull and again at the shoulders. An oversize pillow forces

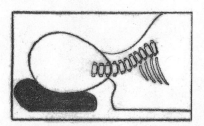

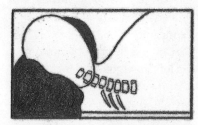

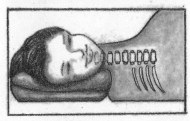

your neck up; it either hangs in space unsupported or twists sharply to make contact with the bedding.

Beware of bowl-shaped pillows with center cutouts for the skull that tend to lock the head in place. Oversize pillows can have the same effect, pinning your head in one fixed position until neck pain and insomnia become almost inevitable. An ergonomic pillow will support your head and neck while permitting movement. The pillow

fills the space beneath your neck, leaving it relaxed and straight. Good neck support at night—could this be exactly what you need to change your life?

Resist the One-Pillow Approach

Don't be stingy with your pillows. Two small pillows mean flexibility and better support. Ultra-soft down yields more easily than anything else.

The Full-Body Pillow

Placing a full-length body pillow between your knees and elbows provides support for the bony parts of your body, an ideal setup for thin individuals or anyone whose legs and arms become numb at night. This is an essential ergonomic tool if you are pregnant or need to bolster your arms and knees in the side-lying position.

Test your pillows and mattress together; they don't work properly separately. Good pillows provide just enough support to keep the head level. Remember, the human body is never comfortable for long in a static position. You must be able to move your head easily during sleep.

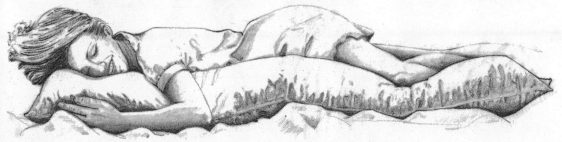

Bed Making in Thirty Seconds

Your own body can be your worst enemy in bed. As sweat and bits of cast-off skin accumulate, the bed becomes an unhealthy place and your sleep patterns suffer. If you don't want to wrestle with a pile of bedding every night, consider eliminating it. The ergonomic solution, substituting a completely enclosed comforter or *duvet*, for the traditional pile of blankets, feels good all night long.

Place the comforter inside a cover (see illustration) made of high-quality cotton, like damask, which has a sensual texture. The cover surrounds the comforter in much the same way that a pillow case fits around a pillow. Once it's enclosed, the comforter actually replaces the traditional top sheet and blankets. This simple change also aids cleaning, bed making and sleeping itself. With the duvet, no part of your body touches material that cannot easily be laundered.

Down feels great because of its loft, an ergonomic feature that insulates without adding weight. But down easily loses its loft when laundered, which makes it unsuitable for the very young. Down can also shed tiny feathers and dander, which create allergy problems for sensitive individuals. Before you invest in a down duvet, borrow one for a week and see how your nose likes it. Artificial polyester down is hypoallergenic, washable and nearly as lofty. Comforters filled with silk and wool are expensive and difficult to clean. Wool also creates allergic reactions of its own. Cotton provides an inexpensive alternative in warm climates and can be machine washed. However, it lacks the loft and coziness of both real and synthetic down.

A down duvet feels light and airy because it is. Airing your bedding outside becomes a simple matter, and bed making is reduced to a thirty-second procedure. Try a comforter once and you will never go back to separate blankets and top sheets.

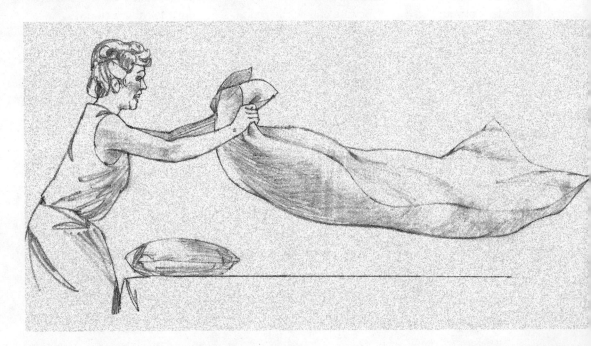

Making a Comforter Cover

Measure your comforter. Your cover should be two inches wider and longer than your comforter.

1. Select two flat sheets or lengths of cotton fabric. Flannel stays cozy in winter, damask is silky and elegant, seersucker remains crisp.

2. Sew the fabric pieces together, leaving a large opening on one side and small hand-size openings at the corners of the other side (as shown).

3. Sew snaps (optional) every ten inches on open side.

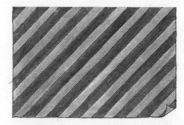

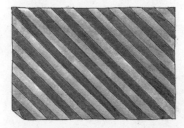

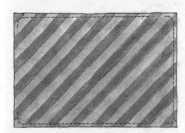

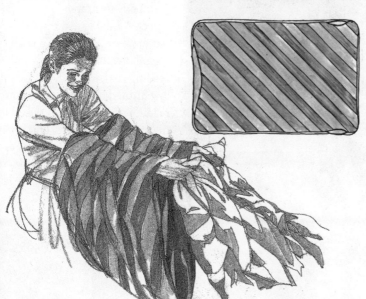

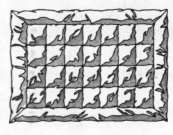

Putting the Comforter Cover on Your Comforter

1. Turn the cover inside-out.

2. Lay out your cover and comforter as shown.

3. Insert your arms through the large opening and pull back on the cover until your hands emerge through the small openings.

4. Grasp the comforter by the corners and pull it through the cover.

5. While grasping the corners, align the sides and corners and shake down the comforter.

When your comforter fills the cover, fling it onto your bed.

How to Read in Bed

At the end of a long day spent suffering the insults of bad ergonomics and rude machines, you have the right to relax in your own bed, to read, and then to dream. So you pick up a book and prepare to unwind. Suddenly you're squinting at poorly illuminated pages, you're uncomfortable and your neck

Avoid lamps with wide shades, which will flood half the room with unwanted light while your reading material remains underlighted. A bed light should be infinitely adjustable and capable of working at various intensities. Choose a light with a built-in dimmer if possible. Make sure the light source itself is well shaded.

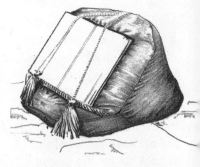

Reading for Hours without Fatigue

Reading in most beds requires that you use your hands, arms, neck, head and legs. And if the book is exciting, you might remain in a single position for hours, which puts a strain on all those body parts. On the other hand, the more relaxed you become, the harder it is to hold the book in place. Lifting your knees helps for a while, but again, you shouldn't have to use the lower half of your body to support a tiny object. A tiltable bed tray helps, but the best solution is a reading pillow. Propping up your reading material with a book pillow immediately improves your reading angle. You don't need to tilt your neck forward, and it also frees up your arms and shoulders from holding the book in place.

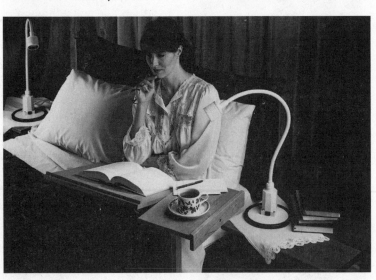

begins to ache. The arm you were leaning on falls asleep. In your last waking minutes, you are confronting yet another ergonomic challenge: struggling to read in bed.

Your Personal Light

Light your bed as carefully as your office. To protect your partner's privacy and to focus illumination on your reading material, you need a narrow-beam spotlight on a flexible neck.

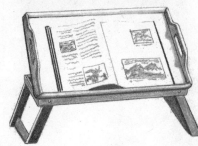

Levenger
420 Commerce Drive
Delray Beach, Florida 33445
(800) 544 0880

96

Privacy in Bed

Every time a machine gets close to your body, the ergonomic question becomes, whose needs come first, its or yours? Understanding precisely what a machine will require from you can spare you some truly nasty surprises. The promising little car radio, with its bewildering rows of tiny buttons and slippery knobs, becomes potentially lethal on a stormy night. A vaguely controlled clock radio exacts a lesser penalty: your good night's sleep.

The Tactile Clock Radio

If you must turn on the room lights to operate a bedside radio, you will be interrupting your rest to satisfy the needs of a machine.

Do an ergonomic evaluation of a clock radio with your eyes closed. Touch it. Get a sense of the way it will feel on your night table. You probably won't do critical listening in bed, so the radio's sound quality is much less important than its tactile features. Look for large, unambiguous controls that can be operated easily in the dark. The shapes and textures of the contols should vary enough for you to feel your way around the dial without flooding the entire room with light.

If you're concerned about low-level magnetic fields (see p. 166), avoid plug-in clock

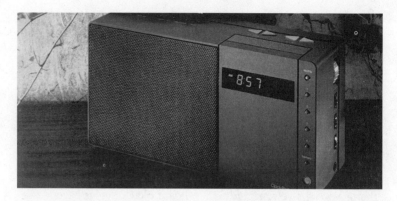

Radio with tactile features

radios with motor-driven clocks (they tell time with moving hands instead of glowing numbers). Digital clock radios, now almost the norm, have eliminated this bedside risk.

Brookstone
1655 Bassford Drive
Mexico, Missouri 65265
(800) 926 7000

Television in Its Place

In a small room your television has no right to a table of its own. No machine that operates by remote control needs to be near your body. Keep precious bedroom space for your-

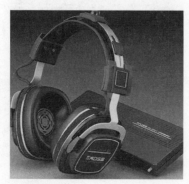
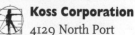

self and hang your television or audio system on a wall. To avoid neck pain, be sure your head is well supported, not tilted backward or forward, when you watch television.

Headphones in Bed

A set of cordless headphones (see illustration) allows your partner to sleep while you listen to a rock concert at front-row volume. You control the volume at the headphones, which operate for many hours on a set of common batteries. A pocket book-size infrared transmitter, fastened to the wall near your music equipment (or sitting on top of it) sends a signal to your headphones. For civilized late-night television viewing in a crowded household, two sets of cordless headphones will operate (at different volumes) from a single transmitter.

Koss Corporation
4129 North Port
Washington Avenue
Milwaukee, Wisconsin 53212
(800) USA KOSS

The Secret Life of Clothes

When a product is manufactured at a factory, its progress is monitored by teams of workers every step of the way. Raw materials and inventory are controlled so excesses don't build up. Think of clothes as the product you must manage. You don't simply buy and wear them; you involve yourself in a complex maintenance process. And your clothes will punish you if you don't acknowledge this. They will pile up in dark corners; they will disappear and turn up long after they have lost their charm. They will take up space you might use for something else. And they will create extra work for you.

As products, your clothes revolve around you in a kind of circle of maintenance. For every hour a garment spends on your back, it will spend days or weeks in various parts of your home. This process, the secret life of clothes, requires an ergonomic storage plan.

The goal: make clothes easy to put away, easy to find, easy to clean and easy to control.

Be Ruthless with Your Garbage

When you find yourself stuffing worn-out socks under a pile of new ones, you have arrived at the moment of truth in your bedroom. What would it take to get rid of the socks? Three steps? Five steps? Before you decide to wait until spring cleaning, ask yourself this essential ergonomic question: Can I afford to organize a useless product? In the bedroom, as in the office, you must be ruthless with your garbage.

Of course, only you can define your own garbage. Whether or not you should hoard old clothes is beyond the scope of this book. However, the ergonomic consequences are worth noting: everything you keep will require maintenance. No matter how organized you are, you will still waste time moving little piles of clothes around and forcing things into drawers where they should fit easily. Never confuse organization, which can create work

where there needn't be any, with ergonomics, which simplifies your life. Keep a goodwill box in your closet and recycle clothes that you no longer want.

The Friendly Closet

Once you are clear on what you actually need, an ergonomic closet becomes the antidote to a chaotic bedroom.

If you dread opening the wardrobe door, if you struggle to jam in each pair of jeans, you probably have too many clothes for a traditional closet with its single hanger rail and shelf. Replace it with a compartmentalized environment containing separate spaces for shoes, sweaters, shirts, skirts and other garments. An ergonomic closet eliminates dead space and lay-

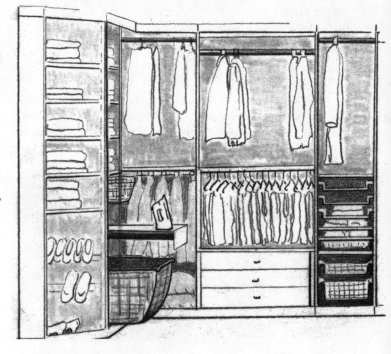

ers of hidden clothes. All storage, from floor to ceiling, becomes visible. Use specialized hangers for accessories.

Clothes Valets

Outside the closet, storage becomes even more haphazard. We are faced with a classic ergonomic challenge: either become obsessive about every article of clothing or live in chaos.

You have a right to relax in your bedroom. When you undress or change clothes, you need a temporary storage place. Without one, garments are draped over beds and chairs, hung on door backs and piled on dressers. They end up wrinkled, mixed up, stacked haphazardly, and even ruined. We've developed this clumsy dependency on furniture as clothes-storage platforms because we no longer have the full-time housewives and servants who once helped us with our clothes. We're still adapting to the modern equitable household in which storage is each person's responsibility. And we have more clothes than people have ever had.

Unmanaged, each garment, every random pile of soiled

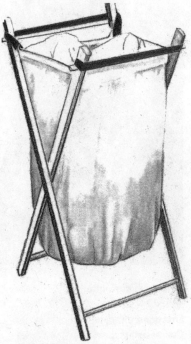

It's 6 A.M.; do you know where your clothes are?

clothes, becomes a land mine of potential stress. If you share a bedroom, you and your partner will like each other more if you have an easy system for storing clothes. The clothes valet, used mostly at the end of the day when you're too tired to hang things up neatly in your closet, brings a new sense of tranquility to your bedroom. Taking up little space, it stands anywhere in the room, ready to preserve an outfit until you find time to return it to the closet. Garments stay clean; pleats and folds remain intact.

This is an evolving product. Most valets include jacket and pants hangers. Ideally, they should accommodate the various needs of men, women and children. Women require fixtures for skirts, handbags, stockings and jewelry. Men need space for pocketed items, suits and ties.

 Winterset Designs
P.O. Box 428
Brattleboro, Vermont 05302
(802) 257 5733

The Washable Hamper

Storage of dirty clothes tends to have a frustrating intermediate stage during which they pile up in a bedroom or closet. A more direct path, from your body to a clothes hamper, makes life easier for everyone. Simply acknowledge that a hamper is a personal item; each person should have one (and take responsibility for managing his or her own laundry). The best hamper is itself washable as well as portable.

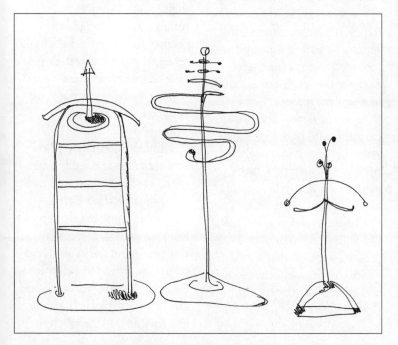

Bedrooms for Allergy Sufferers

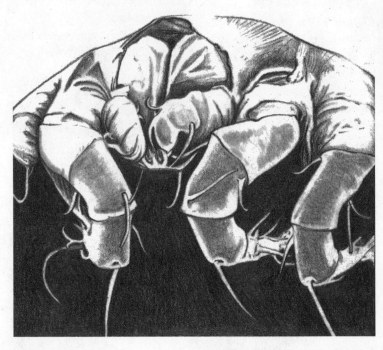

Are you madly pursuing allergy medications while sleeping on the source of your problems? In the bedroom the two most common ergonomic traps for allergy sufferers are low furniture and an innerspring mattress. The day you stop trying to adjust your body to these two objects, you may be able to throw out a drawer full of allergy pills.

The 200 cubic centimeters of perspiration and moisture that are absorbed by your bed every night feed the pinhead-size dust mites that live there. They multiply by the thousands, especially during the winter months, in the mixture of cast-off skin and grime that collects around your bed. They eat dandruff, animal blood (yours) and each other. Their inhaled excrement can cause a range of problems from skin rash to asthma. Allergy pills will accomplish little if you are sleeping in a mountain of toxic debris.

No amount of compulsive cleaning will permanently eliminate dust if you haven't rearranged the bedroom first. Set up the whole room to meet the needs of your body, not the other way around. Be sure every piece of furniture in the room, especially your bed, stands high enough to vacuum and mop under easily.

A dense foam mattress with

Household dust mite
Size: 0.2 – 0.4 mm.
Eats dandruff, dead skin.
Causes asthma, nasal
irritation, itchy eyes.

washable covers eliminates one of the most insidious dust traps: the mostly hollow innerspring. Think of a box- or innerspring-mounted mattress as a large dust box that puffs out clouds of allergenic material every time you lie down. Remove any carpeting and rugs larger than a washable mat. Avoid bookcases, upholstered furniture, dust-gathering knicknacks, curtains and wall-to-wall carpeting.

Choose a solid wood or metal bed with sturdy legs. Avoid pressed wood or fiberboard, which can release formaldehyde and other nasty chemicals. Cover pillows and comforters with regular cotton, not varieties

treated to eliminate ironing which often contain allergenic substances that are emitted over the life of the fabric. Be certain to launder all fabric.

Washing bedding frequently in hot water kills dust mites (mites washed in cold water seem to thrive on the salts in the detergent). But truly effective mite control means finding a way to clean every surface that your body comes in contact with.

Eliminate decorative pillows, lacy neck rolls and teddy bears, which cannot be washed, and cover your headboard with removable fabric panels to protect your body. Use a one-piece removable and washable fabric cover that fastens to a runner on top of the headboard. It's softer and cleaner than wood, tiltable and friendlier to the touch.

Beyond the Ergonomic Home

Most likely your home and office habitats have curious parallels. You spend eight hours in bed at home, and in the office you probably spend eight hours in a chair. If you watch television for many hours at home, conceivably you spend as many hours at work staring into a computer screen. You can struggle nightly with piles of household possessions, only to find yourself battling through mountains of information at work the next morning. ❦ Aspects of the home also exist in the office, sometimes in reverse. In the kitchen we stand even though we could be sitting, whereas in the office we sit when we could be standing. ❦ You have a degree of control in your own home that you cannot hope for in the office. You deserve an accommodating home, a friendly place where you can relax and enjoy yourself after work, and it's in your power to create it. ❦ But what about work? If your office environment is hostile, you arrive home exhausted and your home becomes little more than an ergonomic pit stop.

OFFICE

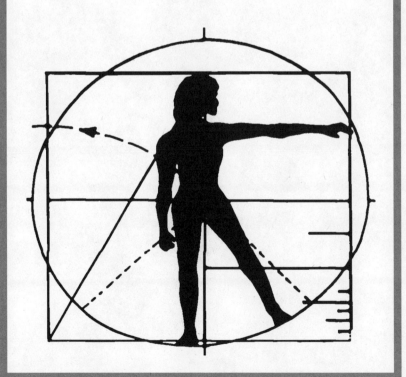

What's Wrong with Your Office?

Y ou struggled with the one-minute manager, but you still fell behind. You got religious about efficiency workshops, and you brainstormed with the company psychologist, but your boss still complains that you're not working up to your potential. ❦ Stop blaming yourself; blame your furniture. ❦ The arrangement of individual work spaces, the layout of office furniture, and even the design of entire office buildings conspire against the people who work within. We cram workers into high-rise buildings, isolating one floor from another. We set up offices in windowless rooms despite compelling evidence that natural light enhances both productivity and health. ❦ Like animals in a zoo we have trouble claiming the office habitat as our own. We become passive, accepting compromises when we should insist on change. Our perimeters begin to shrink. Our personal area moves closer and closer to the desk; we may even give up part of the desk itself. If your dominion ends at the corners of your desk, you will be at the mercy of random noise, bad lighting, pollution, traffic and communication accidents. ❦ You're inside a small cage, looking out.

Your Body in Your Office

Crowding

Noise

Bad air

Traffic

Isolation

Nearly 60 percent of our working population will spend their entire working life in an office. The essential element in the office, the human being, continues to work in an environment that has changed little since the beginning of the industrial revolution. ❦ We know what makes office workers comfortable: features like good lighting, a comfortable chair, good climate control. But psychological comforts such as easy access to co-workers, privacy and a place to concentrate are equally important parts of the ergonomic picture. Most of all, people want an adaptable office environment—one that can change with changing work requirements. Now that most of the monotonous jobs like copying, calculating and collating have been handed over to machines, office workers can concentrate on transactions involving judgment and experience. ❦ Since you probably don't own your own office, you cannot expect to have as much control as you do in your home. But you can make meaningful changes to the inner circle, the area closest to your body, whether it's a workstation or a separate room.

Blame the Furniture

The first step in developing the ergonomic office is to move the perimeters out, to redefine the *edges* of your habitat. Think of the habitat you call your own as having three concentric circles. The largest one, which you probably share with others, extends to the outside walls of your building. The middle, the room you work in, may be communal or private. The inner circle, usually a desk, is a completely personal space, your workstation.

The less control you have over these three circles, the more your health problems begin to multiply. Conversely, people become healthier and more productive when they can influence their own work environment. Use that argument to sell ergonomics to your boss. Also assume you can't do much about your building design, but you are able to rearrange the office layout.

By looking first at the inner circle, the chair and desk—usually the central element of your office—you can get a sense of how extensive the damage to your habitat has become. If you haven't claimed the workstation for yourself, you may have already lost it. And if you've lost control of the inner circle, you probably have no control anywhere else in the office.

You're not alone.

Just as surely as bulldozers advanced on the primeval forest, the most personal part of our office habitat—the desk—is under assault and will be changed forever. And like the spotted owl, the snow leopard and the blue whale, we press on blindly, unable to comprehend the forces that threaten our habitat. First the hunting gave out—we had trouble finding a pen, pencil, crayon, *anything* that would write. (Writing implements once dominated the desk.) Then the territory changed: we stacked papers on chairs and planters, balanced the phone on top of the copying machine and banged our knees on spindly metallic folding-table legs. Fighting desperately for space that was no longer there, we retreated steadily, making excuses for little piles of personal items that littered the rug. Our feet caught suddenly in a tangle of electric cords, yanking the computer off the desk . . .

Because of a single misguided assumption, that our habitat could not extend beyond the edges of our desk, we began to hate going to work.

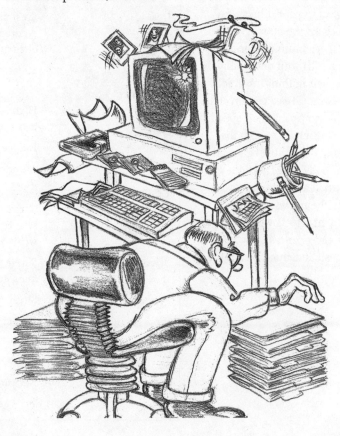

The Office Health Crisis

We cannot know precisely how much nonspecific pain, one of the chief complaints in hospital emergency rooms all over the country, is generated by poor ergonomics. We do understand that painkillers have become a fixture in most offices. When the coffee break yields to the aspirin break, our habitat is destroying our effectiveness.

Pain usually comes from trying to adapt to things as they are in the name of efficiency. Instead of a single serious mistake, you may discover a pattern of neglect in your office, a failure to claim the habitat for yourself. An ergonomic chair that collides with your desk will accomplish nothing. Your job not only requires a certain chair, it should complement a specific desk. Furthermore, both the chair and desk must be keyed to your body. The moment you sit down at a computer workstation, the network of interdependent effects widens. Disk drives and printers crowd onto your desk, locating noise right under your nose instead of across the hall. Suddenly you're staring at a luminous screen for hours at a time, and every light in the room affects you personally. The fax machine and modem stand ready, along with the trusty telephone, but your moods are now at the mercy of electronic communications accidents with people you will never meet.

Your office can punish or help you; the choice is yours. If you're already in pain, don't panic. Use the following list to identify the problems. Begin here to create an ergonomic habitat.

Identifying the Health Problems

Wrong choice here	Leads to
Furnishings	
Chairs	Chronic back, shoulder and neck pain, numb legs, cold feet
Desk	Eyestrain, stress, repetitive motion syndrome characterized by severe pain, often in the back
Storage	Stress, allergies, accidents
Ambience	
Sound	High anxiety, aggressive behavior, inability to concentrate, hearing loss
Light	Fatigue, depression, eyestrain, headaches
Air	Allergies, headaches, drowsiness
Computer	
Keyboard	Carpal tunnel syndrome characterized by severe pain in the neck, shoulders, arms, wrists and hands
Screens	Severe eyestrain, allergies, possible radiation poisoning
Printer	Stress, inability to concentrate
Workstation	Poor circulation and muscle tone, back pain
Communications	
Electronic mail, fax	Aggressive behavior, emotional problems
Telephone	Neck and shoulder pain, stress

6. Territory

For most of us the office is a place where we go to suffer a variety of environmental accidents. Some turn out to be advantageous, even to the point of giving unfair leverage over others. Most of the time, however, they are bad accidents, wasters of time and effectiveness, vitality, health, and motivation."[1] ❦ The further outside the area of your desk you get, the more you need to compromise. The important thing is *to start* exercising some control away from your inner circle. You have ergonomic rights that extend to the outer surface of the building. ❦ Chances are you won't be consulted when the time comes to lay out a whole floor. However, you'll probably have something to say about your own work area and the areas nearby. Here are the ergonomic priorities.

Territorial Ergonomics

Floor layout

Modular office systems

Expandable office systems

Access to tools

Access to people

1. ROBERT PROBST, *The Office, A Facility Based on Change,* Herman Miller, 1968.

Modular Partitions

The term *modular* has become a convenient marketing "hook" used to describe virtually anything that isn't nailed down. A twelve-foot steel bookcase that must be bolted to the wall with special tools cannot be considered modular by anyone but an Olympic weight lifter. Furniture that requires a forklift to move isn't modular. The modular office requires manageable pieces that not only are easy to move and assemble (with normal tools) but can be *expanded* as the need arises. Don't tear down your walls without them.

When the office can be changed readily, work groups that require proximity can be set up almost anywhere. Psychologists have learned that many of the fears, antagonisms and generally negative behavior in organizations arise because people simply do not know what others are doing. In the true modular office, restrictive walls and furniture are movable, and virtually everything can be rearranged.

But the modular office has peculiar organizational pitfalls of its own. In the name of economy, somebody usually figures out that the room can be sepa-

rated into a great many smaller sections. Consequently the modular walls, which were meant to bring freedom, begin to move in on people, locking them into tiny cubicles of noise and visual pollution. Printers buzz, lights flash randomly, people shout across dividers and telephone and electrical cords lurk near every walkway. Once in place, the cramped cubicles are seldom moved.

Set up a modular office correctly and you can transform the lives of everyone who works within. Get it wrong and you create an instant sweatshop.

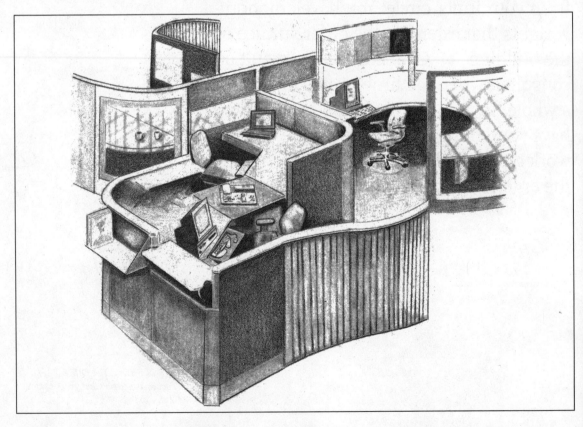

Access to Tools and People

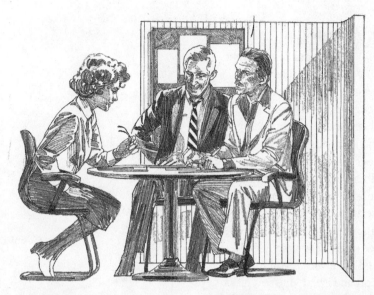

You will get more done if you can see your tools. Yes, this means a certain amount of clutter, but *hidden tools are seldom used.* Consider turning every possible surface into a meaningful visual display. This is your territory, not an art gallery; you owe yourself the most effective and motivational work environment possible.

Use white boards and attractively upholstered panels for bulletin boards. Store useful magazines on slanted display shelves. Tired of digging through a pile of junk every time you need a paper clip?

Modular panels can accommodate tool rails, which are small horizontal racks that keep materials such as tape, staplers and pens in full view (not lost in a drawer) but off your worktable.

Access to People

A personal office, even if equipped with a round meeting table, doesn't necessarily offer the right environment for a small meeting. Blackboards and other communication tools such as slide projectors and overhead viewers aren't practical. Meetings turn an office into a public place.

As work groups are formed to tackle various projects, you will need a place for them to meet. Set up your walls to create small, conveniently located conference areas for frequent small meetings. Small meeting areas can also serve as havens for people who need to escape for awhile from a private office but want to continue working.

Partitioning

Modular	Sweatshop
Cubicles are sized according to task.	As many cubicles as possible are crammed into a space. Larger cubicles are assigned according to status.
Partitions have built-in channels for electrical, phone and computer wires.	Partitions have fixed lighting accessories. Electrical wires are taped to the floor or left loose.
Partitions accept tool racks, vertical storage and display storage.	Partitions cannot be modified.
Height, texture and color of panels can easily be changed.	One type fits all.
Transparent panels for people in intensive communication jobs provide both privacy and accessibility.	One type fits all.
Secretary's desk is positioned behind tinted glass partition.	Secretary's desk is in the hall way, unprotected.
Adjustable task lights are installed.	People struggle to adjust to built-in fixed lighting.

Work Space Enclosures

When planning your office layout, consider the inevitable trade-off between access and privacy. You will feel vulnerable and may have difficulty concentrating with no enclosure at all. Simply adding a solitary wall behind your back increases your feeling of security. You will be most comfortable when enclosed on three sides. When completely boxed in, however, you may feel cut off and isolated. Use a glass wall to create a sense of physical safety while preserving visibility and contact with events outside your work space.

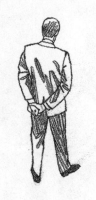

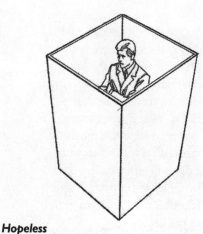

Hopeless

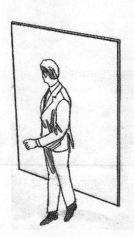

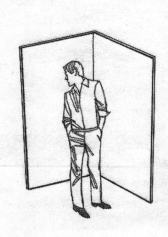

Acceptable

Preventing Traffic Accidents

Will people be shouting across your desk? Are entrances, elevators and corridors insulated from work areas? Evaluate the potential for communication traffic accidents before you set up partitions for the first time. When experimenting with traffic options remember: proximity encourages communication.

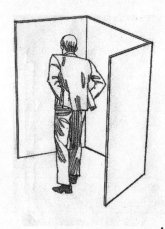

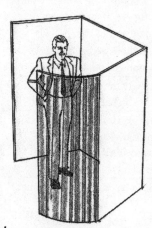

Useful

7. The Inner Circle

Sitting down at your own desk, surrounded by reachable and familiar tools, you are in the inner circle of your office. Every ergonomic improvement here will create tangible benefits for you all day long. ❦ At the heart of the inner circle, the most personal spot of your entire habitat, is the chair. Nearly everything you do will be managed from this point. The chair must fit you perfectly; compromises will cost you dearly. The right chair can transform your life, while the wrong one will turn you into a bundle of aches and pains. You are what you sit in. ❦ The desk has become an ergonomic battlefield on which office workers are steadily losing territory. To reclaim it, you must prepare yourself to do battle with your office tools. Think of your desk as a completely private part of your habitat, *every inch of which is already taken up by your needs.* ❦ Your desk and chair are interdependent parts of the habitat; choose them together. The desk defines a habitat as an office; a chair makes it livable.

The Art of Sitting

The human body is built to move, not sit. Nevertheless, on the farm, in the factory, and especially at the office we're getting more work done by spending more time seated. In fact, with every gain in productivity there seems to be less need to get up and move.

Say what you will about your fabulous new computer, but studying that luminous screen forces you to remain in an even more rigid position than the typewriter did. And the computer is indefatigable. By providing a never-ending stream of instant feedback, it encourages you to tolerate a stiff neck and burning eyes rather than leave some little task undone. Hours go by while you press close to a flickering screen, squinting.

What Is Your Job Doing to Your Back?

Gradually, your body begins to pay a terrible price. More time is lost to backache than to any other malady except the common cold.[1] So the ergonomic question becomes, what is a full day at your job doing to your back?

Perhaps the backaches have already begun. Your neck and shoulders may be so perpetually tight that bad moods surge from one day to the next. Take heart. All of your problems may be caused by spending eight hours a day at a fancy computer while sitting in a broken-down chair. If you're hurting, an ergonomic chair can dramatically change your life.

1. Arbetarskyddsnämnden & Brevskolan, "Ergonomi," Stockholm, Sweden, 1979

Standing is easier on your back than unsupported sitting, and sitting with dangling arms is easier than typing.

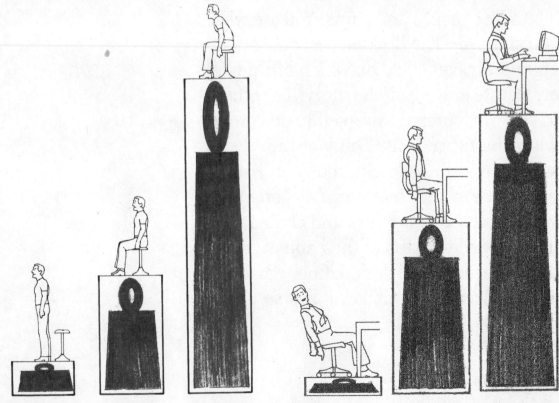

The Basic Ergonomic Chair

Unfortunately, the word ergonomic is bandied around by far too many chair manufacturers. Before you choose a chair, it's worthwhile to think about what actually works—and what doesn't.

Traditionally, the ordinary typing chair had more ergonomic features than any other office chair, but it also had its problems. It could be adjusted, but only if you were willing to get down on your hands and knees. Usually, a typist made a stab or two at the controls before tightening down the bolts a final time and "adapting" to an "average" setting. Most typing chairs lacked an armrest, an important ergonomic feature in almost any chair. Also, since typing chairs were built for women, larger men had trouble fitting into them. Nevertheless, with all its faults, the early typing chair did manage to provide rudimentary

Adjustable Chairs

Whether you're doing computer work or simply going through your in box, you're probably already looking at adjustable chairs. Adjustments, however, are virtually useless unless they are easy to do. Otherwise you won't bother making them. An ergonomic chair must be adjustable as effortlessly as possible in four critical ways:

1. Height
The seat height above the floor can be changed.

2. Back support
Support can be aimed at the actual curve of the lower (lumbar) back.

3. Pelvic angle
The angle of the entire seat can be tilted.

4. Arm support
The armrests can be adjusted vertically.

support for the lower back as well as offer a clumsy way to adjust the overall height of the chair. Some of the most expensive office chairs available today do not include these two essential features.

The Executive Chair
Bristling with polished wood, leather and brass, the executive chair can easily turn into an ergonomic disaster. Status-conscious designers insist on adding an extra foot or two to the top of the seat back, but this extra height conveys a regal impression at the expense of the executive's health. A high-backed chair pushes the upper back forward while forcing the lower back to bend backward. Borrowing an idea from certain luxury cars, many executive chairs are actually designed with a soft *cavity* to accommodate the distended lumbar back, a terribly cynical approach to seating design.

The Knoll Group
105 Wooster Street
New York, New York 10012
(212) 343 4000

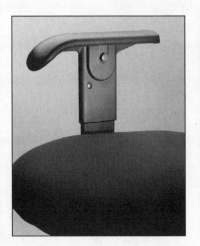
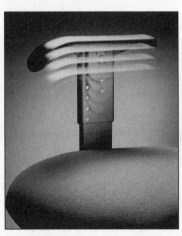

If your chair doesn't support your arms all day, you will.

Using Your Body to Choose a Chair

Make a list of every job you do while sitting, then answer these questions:

Is the chair comfortable . . .

With shoes and without?
With high and low heels?
With your feet on the desk?
With the keyboard (if you use one) in your lap?
While leaning back with your arms behind your neck and looking out a window?
With your legs crossed?
If you get in and out of it quickly?

Does the chair . . .

Move smoothly and easily while rolling around the floor?
Easily adjust while you are sitting in it?

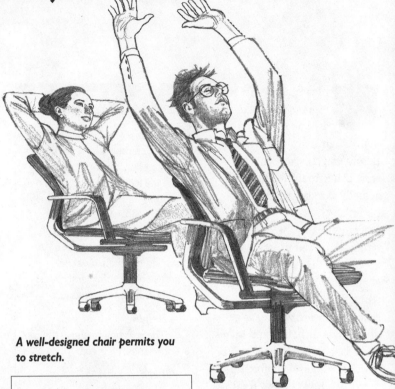

A well-designed chair permits you to stretch.

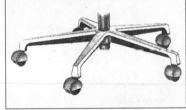

Five spokes permit you to move and remain stable.

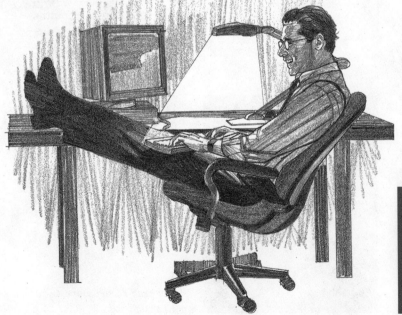

"I have discovered that all human evil comes from this, a man's being unable to sit still in a room."—BLAISE PASCAL, *PENSÉES*, 72

Ergonomic Checklist for Chairs

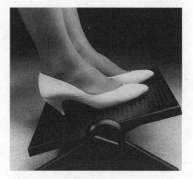

True lumbar back support

Critical. Maintains the natural curvature of the hollow of the back.

Waterfall edge

Prevents numb legs, cold feet, varicose veins and excruciating late-night calf cramps by relieving pressure on the blood vessels of the midthigh. The forward edge of the seat must slope downward gently. If you can feel it pressing against your thigh, it's too high.

Padding

Less is more. Too much makes it difficult to get in and out of your chair and defeats other ergonomic features.

Mobility

The chair should roll effortlessly. Five-spoked bases make it much safer.

Armrests

Allows your chair (instead of your upper back) to support the weight of your arms while you work. Offered as an option on most office chairs. A well-designed armrest does not extend out in front of the chair.

Depth

Too much can be a problem for the small individual, especially in executive chairs. With your back well supported there should be just enough room for a closed fist between the edge of the chair and your knee.

Height

Make sure it's just high enough so your thighs make a ninety-degree angle with your lower legs while your feet make a ninety degree angle with the floor. Consider a footrest if the chair is too high.

Footrest

This is an acceptable compromise while working at a high desk or on a chair that can't be lowered. Simply supporting your feet helps to restore the natural curve of the back. Never let your feet dangle in the air. A footrest will limit your mobility. Use a long one that permits healthy squirming.

North Coast Medical
187 Stauffer Boulevard
San Jose, California 95125-1042
(800) 821 9319

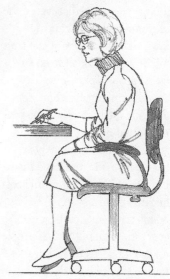

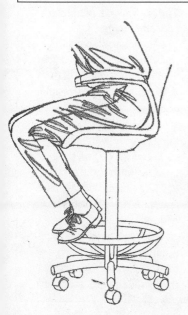

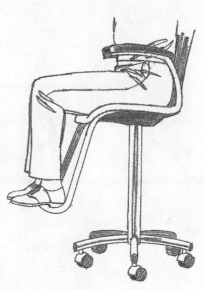

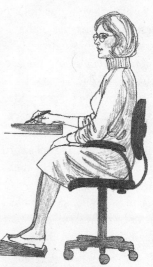

A footrest equals comfort, but the metal-ring type (far left) can impair circulation.

Meetings: How to Sit

People need to do some squirming during a meeting; the question is, just how much? Since there's no need to type or write extensively, the chairs need not be fully adjustable. Silicon Valley scientists of the early seventies thought they had discovered the ultimate meeting chair in the lowly bean bag. Free at last from the limitations of all fixed surfaces, people sprawled with abandon in any direction, certain that the body would be well supported no matter how they landed. By the time the bean bag chair made it to large meetings, the hidden ergonomic cost became painfully apparent: beans crunched loudly with every movement. Also, if people remained perfectly still, it was far too easy to fall asleep.

Assuming your meetings are reasonably short, the chairs need not have as many ergonomic features as the one you sit in all day. However, without lumbar support and a waterfall edge your guests will fidget on their chairs. A self-articulating back as well as arm supports add a generous measure of comfort.

The chair should not have casters, or it will collide with neighboring chairs. Stackable chairs will work in meetings as long as they have the essential lumbar support and a waterfall edge.

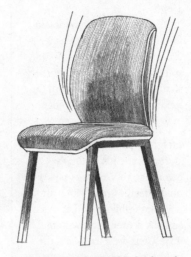
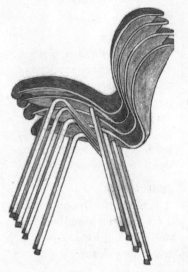

Basic ergonomics: flexible back and waterfall edge

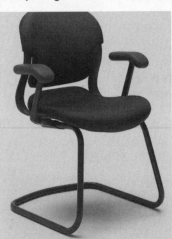
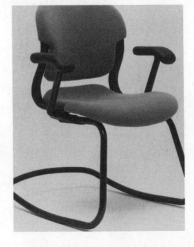

Left: Choose a sled or rocker base for your guests.

 Herman Miller
Zeeland, Michigan 49464
(616) 654 3000

Don't Sit, Walk

The body works better with constant change.

Remember; since you are probably much more sedentary than the office worker of the past, you must pay more attention to your body if your health is to remain intact. Do something nice for your body.

Take a walking meeting.

Have lunch at the gym.

Have a picnic lunch—meet and solve your problems in a park.

Don't be surprised if your group's productivity is higher than it usually is during the traditional sit-down meeting.

Personal Chair, Public Chair

With a minimum of fiddling, a personal ergonomic chair must properly support the body in whatever position you find most comfortable. Generally, you will set it once and forget it, but if you need to make a change, it should be effortless.

A Personal Chair

Chair height, back support and seat-pan tilt should be easily changeable with fingertip controls while you are seated. The best chairs have three-way *adjustable armrests* that maintain crucial support for your arms, neck and shoulders, plus variable seat sizes keyed to male and female body types. The personal ergonomic chair can literally be fine-tuned to your body. Any chair feels good for the first ten minutes. A personal ergonomic chair will feel good ten years later.

Public Chairs

Most people will resist making adjustments to a chair that will be used by others. Solve this problem with a self-articulating chair that will keep your guests remarkably comfortable without asking them to do a thing. These make ideal meeting chairs simply because they flex responsively with the sitter's body. Whether your guest is bent over a desk or leaning back with his or her feet up, a self-articulating chair will support the whole body in ways that must be experienced to be believed.

Clad in soft fabric, without a single ugly surface or unfriendly part, the best self-articulating chairs are lovely to touch. You experience sitter friendliness.

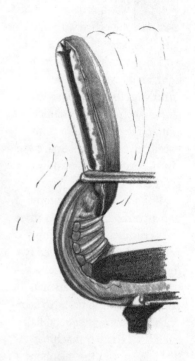

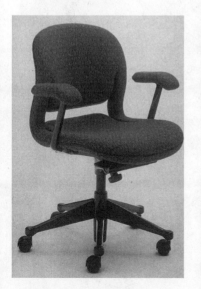

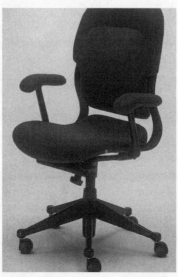

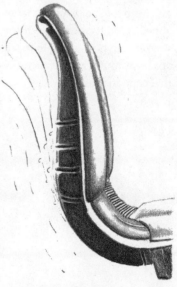

Left, the high- and low-backed personal chair, and, above, the self-articulating chair that moves as you move

Desk Wars

Not long ago the desk was a modest part of the office with few demands placed on it. An office worker made do with a small light, an inkwell and a set of writing quills. If the desk was gloriously free of mechanical clutter, the office was a slow-paced, friendly place. Space was given, never denied—and work proceeded at a snail's pace.

With the advent of automation an army of electronic office tools crowded onto the empty desktop. Noisy mechanized typing and calculating machines—the ancestors of the personal computer—came first. No sooner had the computer established itself than smaller machines to dial and answer the telephone and keep track of appointments appeared on the desktop. Office workers are now trying to make space for much larger machines that copy and fax.

The typewriter, telephone and calculator became indispensable almost the moment they were introduced. Miniaturization helped preserve a little desk space here and there, but the sheer number of accessories rose every year. Scanners, shredders, and laser printers crowded into the office with the usual irresistible allure: use them and your life will be easier.

It was. The machines became indispensable. *But where were they supposed to go?* The desk acquired shelves, flaps, compartments and wings and then overflowed.

The battle for office space was lost on the desk, and when the smoke cleared, the office machine had become more important than the office worker.

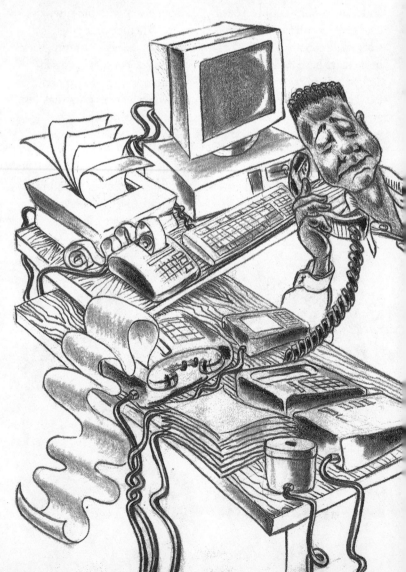

How to Choose an Ergonomic Desk

Is your desk giving you a headache? Furniture stores are bursting with inexpensive, prefabricated white desktops that are meant to complement identical white book cases, file cabinets and chairs. Evaluate a white desktop next to a matte gray one. Note the feeling of tangible relief you feel when shifting your eyes from bright white to a soothing gray.

A white or glossy surface creates glare. If you work in a bright room, your white desk will throw light directly into your face all day long. The ergonomic choice, matte gray or beige, absorbs the light, softening it as it's dispersed.

Generally, the desk surface was better a century ago, when natural woods were favored. Natural wood colors are close to ideal as long as the final finish isn't high gloss.

How Big Does It (Really) Need to Be?

Think of your desk as a workbench that can be divided into separate areas for different jobs. Don't be limited by the rectangular shape of commercial furniture; you can easily combine several tables to create a personal desk with sections on your left or right or to the rear.

To find out how much space you actually need, simply reach out from your original workbench. If you can't reach a spot while swiveling on your ergonomic chair, you're not going to make good use of it. What begins as a U shape with you at the center can become a kind of open-ended polygon that is determined by the reach of your arms, not by the limitations of boxy, rectangular objects. If you need more space, expand, first in a semicircle.

Ergonomic features: rounded end for meetings, vertical storage space, bulletin board and plenty of surface space

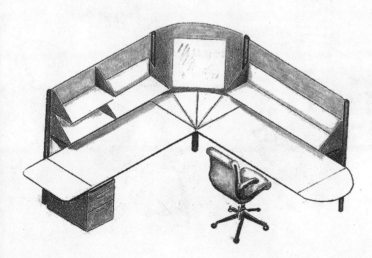

(see Computer Workstation, p. 172)

Basic Ergonomics

The best desk shapes

HORSESHOE: one person; the shape of your reach

ROUNDED CORNER: personal meetings

ROUND: small groups

OVAL: large groups

Ideal desk height

SIT-DOWN: check the clearance envelope for leg and posture comfort

ADJUSTABLE: for computer work (see Computer Workstation, p. 172)

STAND-UP: long, wide jobs, postural variation, quick meetings

COUNTERTOPS: brief transactions

Desk surfaces to avoid

REFLECTIVE: hazardous to your eyes

HIGH CONTRAST: slows you down

ROUGH OR ANGULAR EDGES: hard on the wrists, a recipe for carpal tunnel syndrome (see p. 152)

Using Desk Space

Now that desk space has become such a precious commodity, designers evaluate the area that a desk accessory actually occupies by measuring its footprint. This is the precise space that the bottom of the accessory actually takes up on your desk. Thus, a computer with an eighteen-inch screen that rests on a twelve-inch base would have a twelve-inch footprint, while a mouse or pointing device, which needs to move freely across the desk, has a footprint several times its actual size.

Machines leave footprints on your desktop as they advance toward you. Every inch that's dedicated to a desk accessory is no longer available for you to write on or rest your arm.

The Clearance Envelope

The total amount of legroom you will need under a desk, known as the *clearance envelope,* should allow several inches of movement in all directions. Although you may be able to extend your legs straight out, a desk is useless if it puts pressure on the tops of your thighs. The most critical ergonomic measurement when seated is the amount of clearance between the highest points of your thigh. To check that you have enough space, cross your legs under your desk. You should be able to do so without hitting any part of the desk. You won't be comfortable at a desktop that's too low.

Your Desk as Meeting Place

The way you use your desk immediately sets the tone of a meeting. Want a congenial, friendly chat? Find a way to come out from behind your desk. If space is limited, simply talking across the corner of your desk is friendlier than hiding behind a large table. In larger offices, leave room in front of your desk for a round table to use for casual, relaxed meeings.

Distance makes hearing and eye contact more difficult. Move closer if you want to communicate on an equal basis—but not too close. Too much intimacy can interfere with the effectiveness of your meeting. People become guarded when shoulders and thighs actually touch.

If your guests need to twist their necks in order to see each other, they are probably sitting too close.

The shape of your table also helps to set the tone; rounded corners are friendlier than sharp edges. Use small round tables (or even the rounded end of a desk) to make small meetings in individual offices more inviting.

Do you want to get rid of intruders or people who waste your time? Running a meeting from behind a massive desk communicates distance and rank, particularly if your visitor is seated lower than you. If you have an unwanted visitor in your office, stand up behind your desk. Better yet, meet the visitor at the door and remain standing in the doorway. You need not say a word about how busy you are. This simple technique is guaranteed to keep a meeting short.

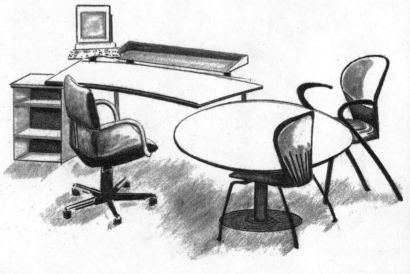

Stand-Up and Modular Desks

Painters, teachers, designers, draftsmen and supermarket checkers use stand-up desks simply because their job typically requires a large work area that cannot easily be reached while seated. A cook stands at a counter for the same reason: kitchen work requires mobility. Getting out of a chair each time to rinse a dish or take a pinch of salt would be annoying. Although we stand while cooking, in the office we remain resolutely seated. We think of white-collar jobs as sit-down work and have come to believe that standing is demeaning.

The ergonomic questions are these: Do you get up from your desk constantly? Are you sitting when you should be standing at your job? If you find yourself checking reference books or working with blueprints, maps and layouts, think about a second desk that permits you to work while standing and provides variety for your body.

If your work involves exchanging paper, exhibits, files and photographs, a standing-level transaction desk on an office divider will significantly boost your productivity and make each job more pleasant. As a second desk it is particularly effective for receptionists and librarians. Also, stand-up desks help keep meetings short and to the point.

The Modular Desk

A modular system can easily include both a stand-up and a sit-down desk. Look for softly rounded edges on all surfaces that you come in contact with and a channel for power and telephone cords. Eliminate power cord tangles (see p. 84). Some desks permit you to plug equipment into the desk itself, using built-in outlets. You then plug the desk itself into the wall.

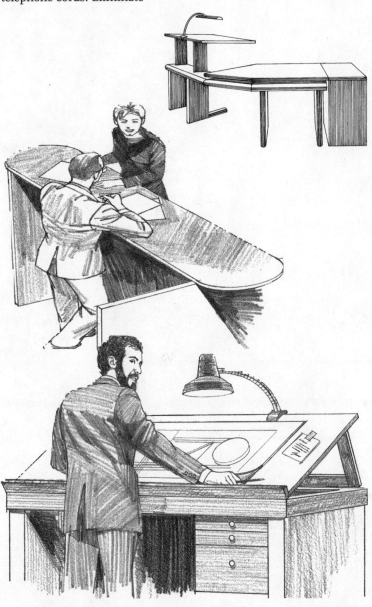

8. Ambience

Ergonomics provides the missing link in the modern health equation: control over the external environment where health problems originate. Paying attention to your body in the name of health—the approach favored by so many fitness books—accomplishes little if you live and work in a hostile environment. We have definite tolerances for temperature, noise and pollution, and we suffer when they are exceeded. ❦ The ambience of your office —the quality of the air, light and sound— affects you all day long. Taking control of it often makes the difference between a dull, aching body and an alert, rested one. ❦ If stress-induced health problems have already begun, look closely at your office environment before you reach for an aspirin. You may only need to change a single item—say, the ventilation near your desk or the positioning of noisy machinery—to bring a tangible sense of relief.

Room Ergonomics

Air conditioning system
Ambient light
Task light
Balanced lighting
Sound enclosures
Sound pads
Sound baffles

The Air

The largest part of your habitat is the air you breathe. Remember, your habitat extends to the outer walls of the building. Make sure you know where your air is coming from and what measures have been taken to keep it clean and fresh.

Stale or polluted air creates a host of unpleasant symptoms that will undermine everything else you try to do with this book. Unfortunately, cleaning up your air is not always a simple matter. In larger offices you may need to make changes to a centralized system. Organize, if necessary, and obtain the support of management to get the job done. Everyone in the building will share the benefits.

Headaches and Drowsiness

Without adequate ventilation, exhaled carbon dioxide builds up in the air; the people in a room create their own air pollution. The larger the group, the sooner your headache will begin. Other airborne contaminants—smoke, dust, chemicals—have nowhere to go, so they accumulate too, adding to your problem.

Irritation

After headaches, the eyes, nose, throat and lungs begin to bother you. Prime culprits include ozone given off by copiers and cigarette smoke.

Allergy and Infection

Airborne dust or chemicals can cause problems ranging from mild allergies to severe asthmatic reactions. Dusty or moldy files and papers release contaminants into the air every time they are handled. Mold and spores can contaminate poorly

Four Steps to Clean the Air You Breathe

1. Allow more fresh air

If your windows are sealed or if noise is a problem, open dampers wide. If your air is supplied through a ventilation system, increase the speed of intake and exhaust fans if possible.

2. Servicing

Make sure filters in the ventilation and air-conditioning systems are regularly replaced and system parts where molds or microorganisms can grow are routinely cleaned and sterilized.

3. Eliminate chemicals

Whenever possible, replace hazardous office chemicals with less hazardous ones.

4. Exhaust fumes

Move machines that use chemicals away from the center of your habitat. Provide them with their own exhaust that is not recirculated with your office air.

maintained air conditioning and humidifying systems, causing a progressive allergic reaction known as *humidifier's lung,* which can lead to scarring and permanent lung damage. Bacteria and viruses that thrive in poorly maintained air-conditioning systems have caused officewide epidemics of flu symptoms such as fever, headache and muscle pain.

Clean Air versus Recycled Air

Portable electric air cleaners remove some airborne contaminants by recirculating stale air through a filter. In the end you get stale air saturated with carbon dioxide minus, say, cigarette smoke. Open a window and the air cleaner stops working properly. Remember, a portable air cleaner may clean up a local problem, but it cannot supply fresh air. Good ventilation *replaces* stale air with fresh air, a more effective solution.

Light: Your Eyes or Your Job?

The ergonomics of lighting has acquired a new urgency because the older working population, which increases yearly, is slowly being driven blind by hopeless office lighting. Meanwhile, the

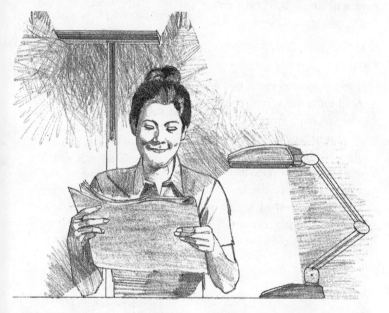

Strong task light balanced by indirect ambient light

personal computer (now virtually a fixture in the office) threatens to finish off the eyesight of the rest of the workforce.

Health Risks

First, the most common blunders: Simply flooding a room with light does not automatically make it a suitable place for human beings to work. Plastering the ceiling with banks of glaring lights creates a warehouselike atmosphere that everyone instantly dislikes. The most conspicuous mistakes bring on problems immediately;

few irritants will degrade your day-to-day health and productivity faster than too much glare or shadow on your work surface. A poor lighting *source* can be less obvious and easier to rationalize. If the sun blasts a wall opposite your desk for a few hours or the antique lamp you treasure glows brightly in your computer screen, you press on heedlessly, not realizing that sloppy lighting will teach you the limits of your body the hard way.

How Light Affects Mood

Aside from making everything more realistic, natural light has some surprising health benefits. Studies of regions with dark winters have demonstrated

that light deprivation can create distinct health problems like depression and weight gain. The afflictions begin to vanish as the days grow longer, disappearing altogether by the summer solstice. The problem, known as seasonal affective disorder (SAD), points the way to an important ergonomic principle: too little light is actually dangerous to your health. Take the SAD Light Test (see next page).

Working in a poorly lighted office, you can experience very real physical problems from simple light deprivation. Light is measured in units called lux. A typical artificial office light provides about 500 lux. (Only 250 lux is recommended for someone working at a computer screen.) Daylight, even on a cloudy day in northern Europe, supplies as much as 10,000 lux, while sunshine close to the equator provides a staggering 80,000 lux. The generally buoyant moods we associate with sunny weather are probably directly tied to simple light exposure. Natural light in your office can easily boost the illumination levels by a factor of twenty or more. Such an increase in levels of light makes a decisive difference in your mood, particularly if you are a SAD sufferer. The ergonomic question is, *how can you control it?*

The SAD Light Test

Is Insufficient Light Making You Depressed?

Do you live in a place that has much less light in the winter than in the summer?

Do you work nights and sleep days?

Do you sleep more during the dark part of the year?

Do you often feel drowsy and have a hard time getting up in the morning?

Do you feel irritable and gloomy in the winter?

Do you feel much better in the summer?

Consider a light box if you work the graveyard shift.

Do you feel lethargic during the darker months?

Does your sweet tooth keep you snacking all afternoon and evening?

If you are a woman, do you have trouble with premenstrual syndrome and related carbohydrate cravings?

Do you gain weight in the winter?

If you answered yes to two or more of these questions, you may be suffering from SAD. Make sure you get more light—ideally natural light—daily. Over a period of a week, exposure for two hours a day to 2,500 lux (the intensity of four or five office lights) completely eliminated SAD-induced

Vision Breaks, Aimless Staring

We take our eyes for granted until we experience problems with them. Then, we have little idea what to do. Taking a break every twenty to thirty minutes to simply stare off into the distance, perhaps out a nearby window, will significantly relieve eye strain. But will your window gazing provoke the boss? You may have to post the Ergonomic Bill of Rights (see p. 186) before trying this. All the better if you can do your staring while taking a walk. The walking meeting, which will boost circulation and keep the back supple, also helps the eyes. Since our eyes haven't changed much since we were hunters and farmers, normal long-distance seeing still provides the most restful position. (For more eye fitness tips see p. 165).

depression and carbohydrate craving in a group of laboratory subjects.[1] Additional light exposure in the morning helps to ensure a good mood throughout the day.

Self Care Catalog
5850 Shellmound Street
Emeryville, California 94662
(800) 345 3371

1 *Scientific American,* "Carbohydrates and Depression," January 1989, p. 68.

Glare and Shadows, Light and Aging

Glare and Shadows

Beware of uncontrolled light sources. We all know not to look into the sun or stare at a bare light bulb for hours, but how many of us will try to do serious work opposite a sunlit window or brilliantly reflective wall? No matter how beautiful your view, you must finally choose between it and your work.

Veiling

Glare lurks in every unshaded window. The moment daylight bounces off a shiny desktop, low-level glare obscures your vision as though a thin gauzy veil were placed between you and your work. As contrast is reduced by the reflected light, you find yourself straining to see, just as if there was too little light instead of too much. The degrading effects of this phenomenon, known as *veiling,* are cumulative. Eye strain and then headaches can wreck your day, all because you have too much light, not too little. Remember, light that's reflected into your face does nothing for you. Veiling is a hidden thief of light in your office.

Trying to work at a sunlit, reflective desk is an uphill struggle. Relentless glare grinds away at your senses. You get tired much sooner, and if you press on, blinding headaches may suddenly bring everything to a halt. The problem is solved not by stockpiling aspirin but by eliminating the sources of glare.

Light and Aging

National Lighting Bureau studies confirm that subjects in their twenties need much less

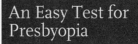
light to perform well than older workers. Higher illumination levels are essential for people over forty.

After forty, most people develop a condition known as presbyopia, which makes focusing sharply on close objects, such as small print, difficult. When the crystalline lens in front of the iris begins to harden, the eye functions more like a fixed-focus camera than an adjustable lens. Sharp images of distant objects are still possible, but those closer than three feet appear dim and blurred. The problem intensifies in dim light, particularly when working with small letters or poor-quality print.

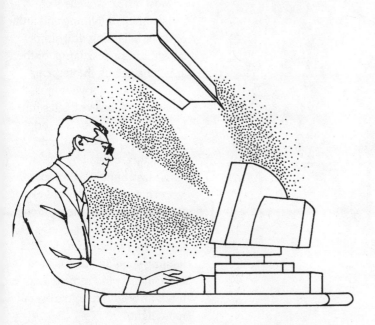

Setting Up Ergonomic Lighting

Generally, you need two kinds of lighting in an office: *ambient,* which provides general illumination, and *task,* which can be tailored to illuminate specific jobs. You must find ways to control both. Begin by asking yourself the question: do I have the right light for my work?

Ambient Lighting

No law requires you to illuminate your office as though it were a hospital emergency room. General lighting can be subtle, pleasant, even enjoyable. Equip your ceiling lights with dimmers and set them up so that small groups of lights can be switched on independently. Each light should also be fitted with a diffuser, which is essential to glare-free illumination.

Ambient lights

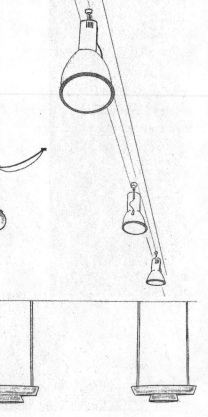

Task Lighting

Trying to make do with ambient lighting that is not actually dedicated to illuminating your work area is a sure recipe for frustration. Truly ergonomic lighting is adjustable both in direction and intensity. Natural light is free but difficult to control. Although uncontrolled artificial lighting can spread glare as easily as unfiltered sunlight, it's much easier to configure to specific tasks. Task lights, designed to illuminate a specific job, should never be confused with movable lamps, purely decorative wall lights or general ceiling lights. A good task light will illuminate your work and little else. Opaque shades will prevent direct light from reaching your eyes.

Balanced Lighting

Most offices provide too much ambient lighting and little or no task lighting. But simply substituting a desk lamp for the annoying ceiling fluorescents won't do much for your eyes. The pupil of the eye dilates in low light and contracts in bright light. Constant dilating and contracting, caused by, say, a single task light in a dim room, is a major cause of serious eye fatigue. Make sure the light on your work area is balanced elsewhere in the room. Task lighting shouldn't be much more intense (no more than five times as bright) than the overall room light.

Controlling Glare

Begin to control glare by making sure that no direct or reflected bright light can reach your eye while you're working. Do a quick inventory of your office: whenever possible, eliminate large, glossy, highly reflective surfaces across from your desk or on the surface of the desk itself. White desktops (see p. 121) are deadly. Use diffused lights for general illumination. If you have north-facing windows, control the natural light

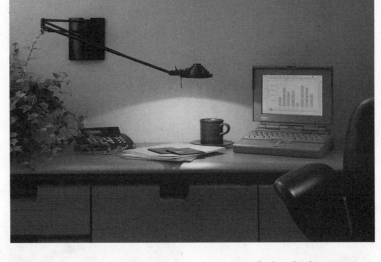

Preventing Eye Fatigue

Eliminate bright or shiny desk surfaces and repaint walls that reflect too much light.

Light-colored ceilings, matte walls, medium-colored furniture and dark floors control glare best.

While you're working

Is the light source visible to your naked eye?

Does the light cause a visible reflection on your work surface?

Is the light source reflected into your eyes until it hurts?

Are shadows cast across your work area?

in your room with semi-transparent sun-reflective shades. Metallic threads on the exterior reflect heat and cut glare. They'll provide far more effective glare control than the old-style Venetian blinds and will also help to insulate the room. Windows that face south, east or west require opaque shades for the direct sun. If possible, position your view facing north to cut down on glare-induced headaches.

Controlling Shadows

Don't try to work with shadows—the worst ones are usually caused by objects blocking a light source that is directly behind you. To eliminate them, move the light source or reposition your desk, whichever is easier. Smaller shadows are usually caused by parts of your body. To prevent your hand from constantly shadowing your work, use a light that originates on the left if you're right-handed or vice versa if you're left-handed. Once you've controlled the *direction* of light you can attend to its quality.

Luxo Lamp Company
36 Midland Avenue
Port Chester, New York 10573
(914) 937 4433

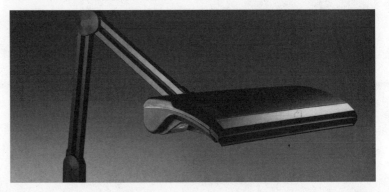

Effective Ambient Lighting

Most ambient light either comes from fixtures in your office ceiling or enters through nearby windows. An ergonomic lighting plan gives you a way to blend these sources or use them independently. Without that essential control, you (and everyone who enters your office) are at the mercy of accidental ambient light.

Equip ceiling lights with dimmers.

Make sure your ceiling light fixtures have diffusers.

Allow sets of ceiling lights to be turned off selectively (vital if you're a computer user).

Consider full-spectrum fluorescents. Although fluorescent lamps were originally a poor choice because of their flicker and cold, bluish hue, full spec-

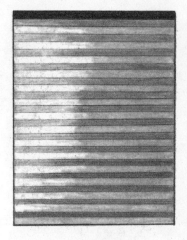

Window shade as diffuser

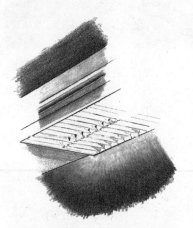

Diffuser for fluorescent light

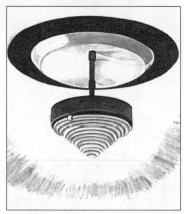

Glass pattern diffuser

trum models represent a significant improvement. Shield them with deep louvers or other diffusers.

Bring in natural light. If you don't have a window, see if you can get one. If you can't arrange for a window, make sure you get enough natural light to remain happy and productive.

IKEA
20700 South Avalon Blvd.
Carson, California 90746
(310) 527 4532

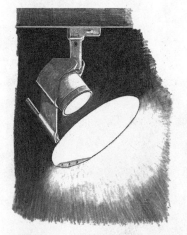

Diffuser for track light

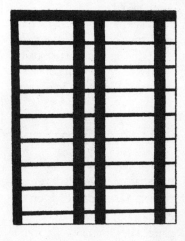

Shoji screen as diffuser

Effective Task Lighting

While ambient lights set the mood in your office, a task light makes detailed work easier. No matter how brightly lit your office is, you will benefit greatly from your own task light. Task lights are reachable inner-circle tools, and you can control them more precisely than ambient lights.

Make each task light movable, so that it can be positioned properly for left- and right-handed workers.

Avoid fixed partition lights. They are annoying at best. A movable task light works better.

The Ergonomic Lamp

Most adjustable lamps fight back when you adjust them. Pull the lamp head two feet across your desk and it moves back two inches. And no matter where the lamp is positioned, every attempt to illuminate your work seems to create serious glare. To further complicate matters, in less than five minutes the lamp becomes too hot

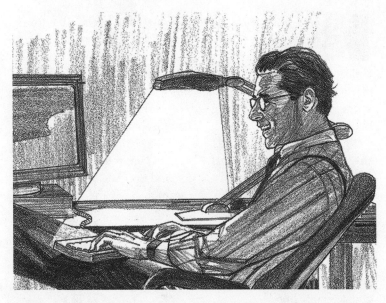

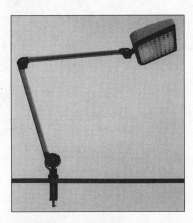

An asymmetrical task light illuminates your keyboard, not the screen.

Task light with diffuser

to touch. You then push it out of your way, "adapt" to a single setting and press on with light in your face.

Adjustments on an ergonomic lamp must be effortless and utterly predictable; the lamp head should remain cool after

hours of use. Look for strong, evenly distributed light that can be directed precisely where it's needed. The newest adjustable lamps provide asymmetrical light distribution and a color-balanced combination of fluorescent and incandescent bulbs. There is no direct eye contact with the light source and no annoying glare.

An ergonomic desk lamp has a way of banishing headaches and eye strain; the moment you turn one on, you can *feel* the difference.

North Coast Medical
187 Stauffer Boulevard
San Jose, California 95125
(800) 821 9319

Bad Noise, Good Noise

Noise continues unopposed because we don't take it seriously. Unlike water and air pollution, which we strive to control, loud sounds leave no lasting damage in the environment.

Nevertheless, noise induces stress just as surely as residual smoke or pesticides; the ear simply cannot adapt to the din of the machine age. The effects of noise are cumulative within the human body. To maintain normal hearing, an individual exposed for a short time to eighty-five decibels, the interior level of a noisy bus, should rest his or her ears for three hours. Moving from a noisy bus to a noisy job literally means adding the noise of commuting time to whatever sound levels prevail in the workplace. Eventually, permanent hearing loss will begin.[1]

There is no cure for most of the damage caused by noise; you must reduce the source. No matter how much attention you pay to other ergonomic ingredients, loud noise will dominate your office habitat and play havoc with your productivity goals. An estimated fourteen million American workers expose themselves daily to hazardous noise levels, often from the machines they use.

Not all noise is bad. A low sound level will shield you from the coughs and outbursts of co-workers and visitors as sirens, braking cars and roadwork lose their capacity to startle. In fact, you can actually use sound to create privacy. Do you want to call home and talk about your children's illness without the whole office offering advice? Or perhaps you must contact your broker, talk to

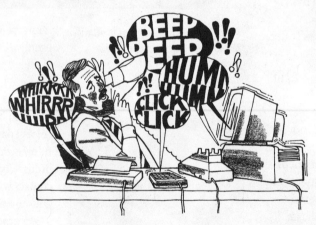

a headhunter or consult with the boss. Overheard conversations are one of the major distractions in modern offices. Good noise occurs in the background and permits you to work without disturbing others. In fact, a completely silent environment drives some people crazy.

Background sound or *white noise* levels should never be intrusive. Ideally, white noise will provide just enough masking effect to hear that a conversation is taking place without actually understanding it.

Unless you want to get seriously involved with rubberized membranes and sealed ventilation systems, forget sound-*proofing*, a technique for eliminating virtually all sound. Unlike light, sound will flow through practically any hole and fill a room. The crack under a door, the electrical fixtures, even the so-called acoustic ceiling (with its inevitable metal lighting cans) provides plenty of spaces for outside sounds to invade your office. Reduce noise, control it, but don't try to eliminate it.

People have different levels of noise tolerance; what's pleasant for one individual may be irritating to another. Since unexpected bursts of noise create far more stress than a constant, high sound level, simply having control over the volume in a room will significantly reduce stress levels.

The ergonomic challenge is to find a way to put sound to work for you.

1. GEORGE BUGLIARELLO, *The Impact of Noise Pollution: A Socio-Technological Introduction,* Pergamon Press, New York, 1976, pp. 387-89.

The Hidden Cost of Noise

Loud sounds at the high and low thresholds of your hearing capability will punish you relentlessly whether or not you actually hear them clearly. In a recent study nearly half of the office workers surveyed mentioned that the comfort they missed most was "a quiet working environment."[1]

Health Risks

Working in a loud room will make you chronically irritable and unable to deal with minor frustrations. Well before you notice any hearing loss, noise fatigue may have become a serious problem. Your blood pressure, heart rate, and metabolism accelerate, slowly at first, then so sharply that the entire body is flooded with adrenaline. Low-level muscular tension spreads through your entire body. Suddenly you're uptight. If the noise persists, a vicious circle begins: tension produces more tension, making relaxation, even at the end of the day, difficult. Worst of all, every one of these sorry effects intensifies as sound levels are amplified. Enough noise, some experts claim, will cause antisocial behavior, even violence.

Most loud noise causes a temporary loss of hearing; the loss becomes permanent when noise recurs frequently. Hearing loss sneaks up on you slowly. The higher frequencies

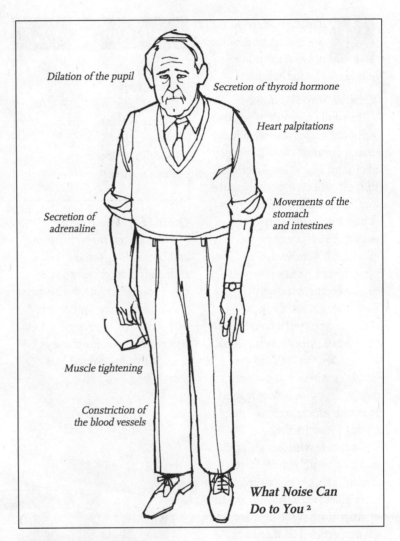

Dilation of the pupil

Secretion of thyroid hormone

Heart palpitations

Movements of the stomach and intestines

Secretion of adrenaline

Muscle tightening

Constriction of the blood vessels

What Noise Can Do to You [2]

disappear first: birds singing, telephones ringing, crickets chirping. When you begin having trouble with conversation, the second irreversible phase of hearing loss has begun. Hearing aids help but tend to perform poorly in places with high ambient noise levels.

1. Steelcase and Louis Harris survey of office workers, Administrative Management, 1980.
2. *Noise Control*, U.S. Department of Labor, OSHA, Washington, 1980.

What to Do about Noise

No matter where you work, start controlling noise at the outer boundary of your habitat.

Weather Strip Windows

Ten dollars' worth of weather stripping may accomplish more than thousands of dollars' worth of custom sound engineering. In most offices, especially those located in older buildings, this is the single most important sound control measure you can take. If your weather stripping is worn or missing, you can be certain that high-frequency sound, the kind that puts your teeth on edge, is pouring in through every crack. Remember, the walls of the building, where you can intercept street noise *before it gets into your office*, are the outer circle of your habitat.

Of course, weather stripping also helps with temperature control, another ergonomic feature. Thick, foam-backed weather stripping has the best acoustical properties. Metal or hard plastic will keep out the weather but does little to stop street noise.

Noise: Quick Fixes

Rugs
Typing pads
Writing pads
Bulletin boards
Acoustic tiles
Padded partitions
Window shades

Quiet Your Whole Office

Hard floors, metal furniture, and bare ceilings make the sounds in a room harsh. The same room furnished with well-padded carpeting, upholstered furniture, fabric-covered panels and window shades conveys sounds that are muted and pleasing.

Move Noisy Machines

With the exception of the automobile, most machinery operates without any kind of sound control. You're expected to adapt to the machine. Use an extension cord or a nearby sound-insulated closet to enforce your ergonomic right to quiet.

Never place noisy machines near corners. The closer your noisy office machinery is to hard noise-reflecting surfaces, the greater the noise it will radiate in your office. With three opposing surfaces, room corners amplify sound noticeably. Move noisy machines to a spot with one reflecting surface, midway between two walls. You will hear the difference immediately.

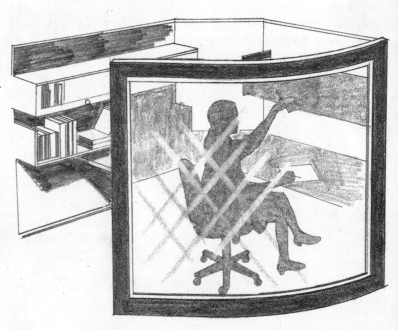

Intercept Noise

Any soft vertical surface provides an effective sound shield inside your office, especially when combined with a sound-absorbent ceiling. High-frequency sound is strongly directional and easily reflected. Bouncing high-frequency sound off the ceiling effectively blocks it before it reaches you.

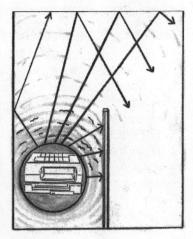

A noisy printer without sound-absorbent ceiling

Set Up Glass Partitions

Divide work spaces with glass partitions that reflect noise without blocking light. People can see each other while carrying on important business privately.

Move Desks Away from Traffic

Passersby are a major distraction.

Silence the Computers

Never take computer noise for granted. Computer manufacturers are just beginning to realize what an enormous difference internal soundproofing makes. This is an ergonomic feature whose time has finally arrived. On older equipment, the fatiguing high-pitched whine of disk drives and internal fans can be significantly reduced by simply placing the devices on thick rubber typewriter pads.

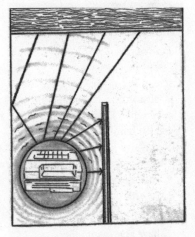

A sound-absorbent ceiling intercepts printer noise.

Silence Your Keyboard

The lowly typewriter used to be one of the noisiest tools in the office. Perfectly silent computer keyboards are now available, although the absence of any auditory feedback may slow you down. Nevertheless, even a "half-silent" keyboard will make a significant difference to those working nearby. You can replace a keyboard without replacing the entire computer.

Use Sound Enclosures

Printers shouldn't be heard. We put up with the typewriter, we tolerate the telephone, but nobody who works near a dot matrix printer can stand its constant buzz-saw whine. Non-impact printers, using laser and ink-jet technology, are virtually noiseless. Until you get your hands on one, put your dot matrix printer in a sound box, which will reduce decibel levels by 90 percent.

Good Noise

The background music used in shopping centers and restaurants provides a kind of white noise simply to keep us shopping and eating. It isn't meant to entertain but to create auditory privacy by supplying just enough sound to mask sudden, annoying noises. The right sounds will also create privacy in your office.

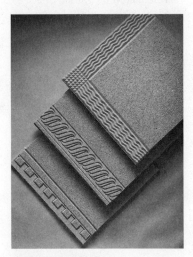

Acoustic tiles

Armstrong World Industries, Inc.
P.O. Box 3001
Lancaster, Pennsylvania 17604
(310) 527 4532

Basic Sound Masking

Although solutions employing good noise are remarkably uncomplicated, people tend to ignore them, hoping somehow to "adjust" to irritating sound levels. Puritanism undermines ergonomics the same way it does all pleasurable experiences in life. Reject the culture of suffering. Allow yourself to enjoy privacy.

Audition Your White Noise

Monitor all noises and keep only the ones that please you. Some are unintentional: the drone of air conditioners or traffic, the hum of voices, even the clatter of keyboards. Others are planned: elevator music or a dedicated white-noise machine. The ideal sound-masking system is never noticed; it brings new peace to the work space and greater privacy. You'll know it's working when you experience a new sense of privacy and a feeling of genuine peace in your work space.

Too Quiet for You?

Do you:
feel that the silence is screaming at you?
always turn on your sound system or television as soon as you get home?
prefer the cafeteria to the library for working on papers?
consider yourself an extrovert?

Did you:
have arguments about keeping the radio on while doing homework? Did you win?
grow up in a loud family?

If you answered yes to several of these questions, consider a personal sound system while you work.

A Personal Sound-Masking System

Take control of the sound in your workplace. A small radio/cassette/CD player may provide just enough privacy for you to be productive. If you find yourself actually listening to the music, it's too loud.

Too Loud for You?

Do you:
often turn down the volume of entertainment systems? If you can't adjust the volume, do you become irritated?
find yourself getting angry and frustrated while trying to work or talk in a very noisy environment?
find that people around you talk too loudly?
have a hard time being heard?
find that people ask you to speak up?
like to be by yourself in a quiet space?

If you answered yes to any of these questions, you will work more effectively in a quiet office. Take control of your office by reducing sound as much as possible. Consider adding soothing white noise if the ambient sounds keep you on edge.

Sound Tools

An inexpensive sound meter takes the guesswork out of noise control. Move the printer, not your desk, and take a reading; hang a sound board, take another reading. Moments after you turn on the meter you know exactly how much noise is penetrating your office, what direction it's coming from and whether or not your sound-control measures are working.

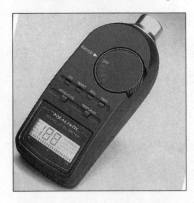

Tandy Corporation
700 One Tandy Center
Fort Worth, Texas 76109
(817) 390 3300

Noise and Your Hearing

A burst of sound above 120 decibels can cause severe pain and permanent damage. The injuries to your body from sound at lower levels are cumulative—jackhammer noise on Friday contributes to the damage caused by a rock band on Saturday. If you are *continually* exposed to noise, this is what you are facing:

Source	Decibels	Effects
Jet engine	120 – 150	permanent damage
Jackhammer	110 – 120	severe noise fatigue and permanent damage
Loud orchestra	100 – 110	extreme noise fatigue
Subway train	85 – 90	noise fatigue; onset of pain; ear protection advised above this level
Car	65 – 75	noise fatigue
Conversation	50 – 60	noise fatigue if nearby
Whisper	30 – 40	no noise fatigue

Source: INGER HULTGREN *Ergonomi*, Esselte Studium, Sweden, 1982.

Then, by flipping a switch, you can tell precisely what kind of noise you're experiencing.

High-frequency sound (printers or appliances) probably originates nearby, unless you're in an older building, while low-frequency sound that pounds your eardrums incessantly (trains or buses) may be penetrating the building from outside.

Room Treatments

Sound baffles are pricey relief for ears battered by throbbing low-frequency sound waves. They turn part of the room into a kind of instrument that can actually be tuned to exclude certain frequencies. This is virtually the only way you can attenuate the very low frequencies (which are *felt*, rather than heard).

Interior Acoustics, Inc.
P.O. Box 839
Bellmead, New Jersey 08502
(800) 221 0580

9. Storage

The physical habitat of the office, filled with furniture and machinery, exists side-by-side with the mental habitat—working in an office, you are paid to think. If furniture supports the body, then storage supports the mind. ❧ As anyone can testify who has seen perfectly competent executives floundering helplessly in oceans of paper, the wrong storage plan can drive you mad. The creative part of office work —problem solving, decision making and negotiating—requires another process that is usually taken for granted: finding and filing things. ❧ Virtually everything done in the office involves getting something and putting it someplace else. Without storage, contracts cannot be signed, suppliers aren't paid, contacts are lost and all business grinds to a halt. If the office is the brain of an organization, storage is its memory. ❧ Any complex human activity requires an ergonomic storage plan to succeed.

The next best thing to knowing something is knowing where to find it.—SAMUEL JOHNSON

Your Storage Rights

The devastating Japanese raid on Pearl Harbor, which provoked the American entry into World War II, owed nearly everything to hopelessly bad American ergonomics. On a lonely outer island hours before the sneak attack, one drowsy sentry actually spotted hundreds of incoming blips on his radar screen. Nothing like that had ever happened before. Was it an equipment malfunction?

Plunging into the radar manuals with one hand on his radiotelephone, he flew through a loose collection of unbound pages and wrinkled addenda. If the relevant instructions hadn't been misfiled, he might have reported bombers instead of birds.

The Guilt-Free Mess

We struggle with piles of paper, eternally stuffing file cabinets with proposals, letters and invoices, knowing that every day's mail will bring a new avalanche. We try, desperately, to become more efficient, if only to keep the desk clear, but we confuse efficiency with neatness. New management techniques, one-minute storage plans and obsessive productivity workshops proliferate. Nevertheless, these strategies fail to produce results.

That some of the most creative and productive people who ever lived worked in utter chaos perfectly illustrates the most fundamental ergonomic storage principle: *you have a right to your own clutter.* Don't be bullied by programs that insist on organizing your whole office (or perhaps just your desk) to fit some preordained model of perfection. The basic ergonomic question is, what kind of storage supports your work style? It's much easier to change your office than your behavior.

Nineteenth-century active storage

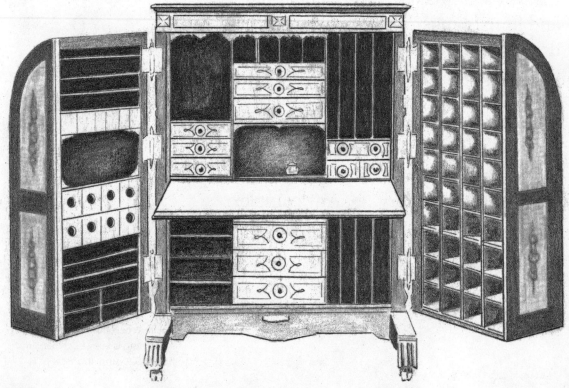

How to Find Things

With an ergonomic storage plan you can become intimate with the most important details of your work, but *only if you become utterly ruthless with your garbage.* Your storage situation is out of control the moment piles of junk begin to dominate the office. Decide work done. Don't be surprised if you run out of space quickly. The trick is to find a way to keep "essential items" from crowding you out of your office

The Knoll Group
105 Wooster Street
New York, New York 10012
(212) 343 4000

Extending Your Brain

One of the less recognized contributions made by computers—with profound ergonomic implications—has occurred recently: access to information without manual searching. By creating a superactive file with a computer, much tedious storage work is eliminated. This ability

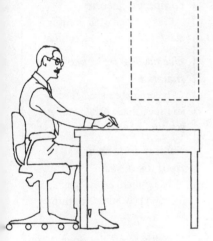

Put available vertical storage space to use.

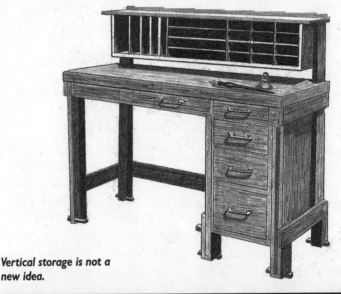

Vertical storage is not a new idea.

what is actually useless and begin to eliminate things.

Setting Up Active Storage

Active storage, as a direct extension of your mental habitat, should stimulate, help set priorities and keep you from missing important appointments. Keep it visible in the inner circle and easily organized. Begin by taking an inventory of the things you actually need all the time to get your

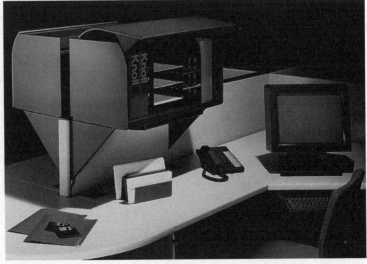

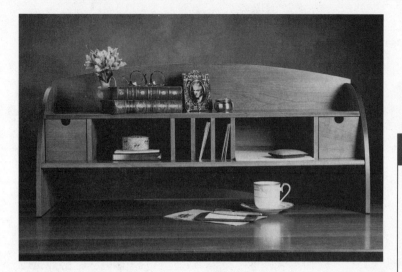

represents nothing less than a genuine revolution in record keeping.

Is your bulletin board overflowing? Computerized "tickler" files set up months in advance take note of important events, then prompt you. Information is kept out of sight (and out of your brain) until the moment you need it.

The early promise of the computer, to bring about the paperless office, was misguided. In fact, it often generates far more paper than ever before. Backing up your files to disk, however, eliminates the need to

Levenger
420 Commerce Drive
Delray Beach, Florida 33445
(800) 544 0880

store paper generated on your computer in the office.

How to Set Up Intermediate Storage

Do you want to eliminate nagging piles of paper from your office? Limit visible storage to your immediate needs and develop a hidden storage plan for items you don't need frequently but want to have handy.

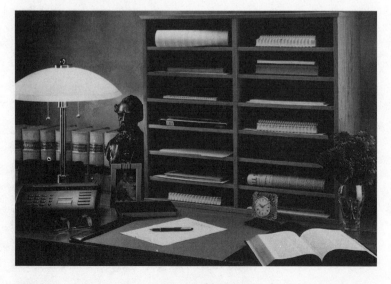

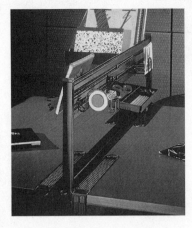

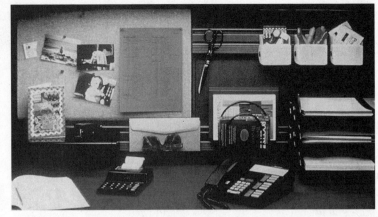

They should be stored in your office but out of sight. If you will need to bend and stretch or use a step ladder, they're too far away.

Beware of the rot factor: papers in intermediate storage have a tendency to age and to become slowly useless.

How to Set Up Long-Term Storage

Long-term storage can preserve government records, prevent a lawsuit or satisfy the IRS. However, *most long-term storage is dead storage.* If you will never need the item again, find the time and courage to discard it—dead storage is use-

less. You will probably find it easier to create a new document rather than fish around for something you filed "just in case" ten years ago.

You may want to keep something because it gives you a sense of security or for purely sentimental reasons. However, since long-term (or *archival*) storage is seldom used, it shouldn't claim precious office space. Perhaps your company has a storage room. If you're working at home, consider a basement or attic.

Herman Miller
Zeeland, Michigan 49464
(616) 654 3000

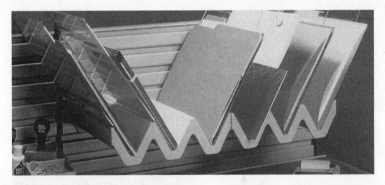

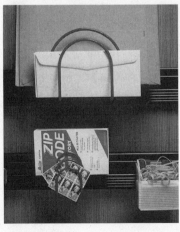

Tool bars keep little items visible but off your desktop.

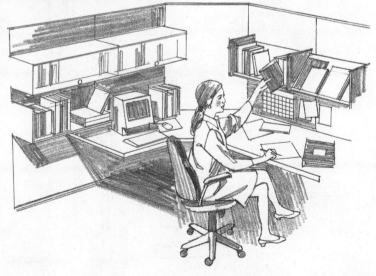

An Ergonomic Storage System

For the chronically disorganized an ergonomic storage system is an antidote to panic. A large, modular unit can combine all of your storage needs in a single wall. Books, art, perhaps audio components and personal items can be displayed on open shelves (as shown) or behind glass doors. Project files at eye-level occupy a space of their own. Attractive wooden doors that close with a satisfying click conceal older files and equipment. Interior shelves roll out to expedite loading and unloading.

The exterior cabinet need not include a single knob, button or exposed piece of hardware. Spring-loaded doors can be set to open and close with the pressure of a single finger. A built-in stand-up desk gives you a way to vary your work routine and provides a handy work surface close to important documents. Electrical cords are routed through hidden channels.

No matter how you set up a wall-size storage system, the effect is one of uncluttered elegance and efficiency. You can leave the system in place for years or take it apart for moving in a matter of minutes.

George Monroe Design
P.O. Box 584
Miranda, California 95553
(707) 943 3094

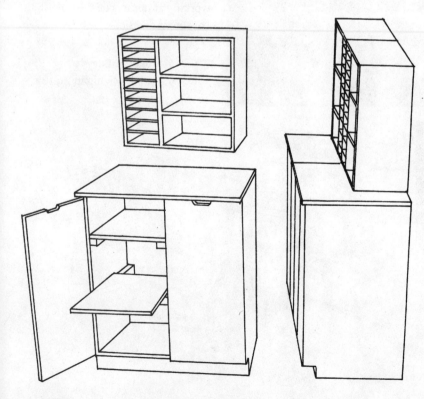

10. The Personal Computer

f you're new to computers, getting one can be the realization of a dream—or the beginning of a nightmare. Few new endeavors depend so much on an accurate understanding of ergonomics. ❦ First the dream: you have a tireless servant, a machine that actually eliminates the need for certain support staff. It can be your proofreader, librarian, financial advisor, stockbroker, project coordinator and newscaster. Using it, you acquire a sense of independence and confidence. Every day you are able to explore new worlds. ❦ It adds little freedoms too: your spelling is corrected, address files are updated and your checkbook is balanced. ❦ At the highest level the computer can transform your life, replacing the post office, eliminating the daily commute and creating flexible work hours. ❦ But take care, the very same computer can turn your job into a distressing ordeal.

Computer Ergonomics

User interface

Laptops

Low-profile keyboards

Keyboard layouts

Mice and trackballs

Wrist rests

Arm supports

Screens and lighting

Screen size

Tilt and pivot screens

Screens and color

Printer speed

Output quality

Paper handling

Disk drives and fans

Cables

Any job that can be done by a machine, should be.
— ARTHUR C. CLARKE, *Profiles of the Future*

Civilizing the Computer

The moment *jobs* are specialized in order to make *computers* more efficient, you commit the classic beginner's ergonomic error—putting the demands of a machine ahead of human needs. When the first wave of computers hit the office, people were immediately divided into ultraspecialized work groups and expected to do a single repetitive job all day.

The word processors (workers assumed the names of their machines) were herded into a word processing center to do nothing but "typing support." Removed from the life of the office and the overall purpose of their jobs, workers became so highly specialized they were unable to do anything but a single computer job. The isolation coupled with the dreadfully sedentary nature of the new job was so demoralizing that nagging stress-related ailments appeared. Performance plunged while absenteeism soared. Anti-technology buffs were quick to blame the machine itself, rather than poor (or nonexistent) ergonomic awareness. The computer, they proclaimed, was indeed a kind of "big brother," keeping track of keystrokes per hour, noting every mistake and timing each break ("you took nineteen extra seconds for your coffee"). It was an evil machine, and with its help the sweatshop

> I saw at once that it was the long-prepared, long-awaited and long feared war between men and machines, now at last broken out. . . . On every wall were wild and magnificently stirring placards, whose giant letters flamed like torches, summoning the nation to side with the men against the machines.
>
> Other placards . . . depicted in a truly impressive way the blessings of order and work and property and education and justice, and praised machinery as the last and most sublime invention of the human mind. With its aid, men would be equal to the gods. The flaming eloquence affected me as powerfully as the compelling logic. They were right and I stood as deeply convinced in front of one as in front of the other.
> —HERMAN HESSE, *Steppenwolf*

had been reinvented.

Although the problems of centralized computer work persist in jobs like insurance claims, telephone directory service, mail-order processing and telemarketing, the unionized worker now has ergonomic protections: mandated breaks built into the day, detached keyboards, glare filters and a host of other features that make the computer a friend instead of an enemy.

Do you?

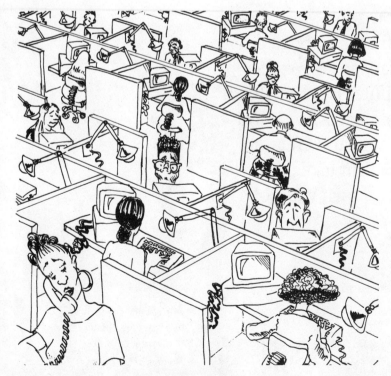

Choosing a Computer

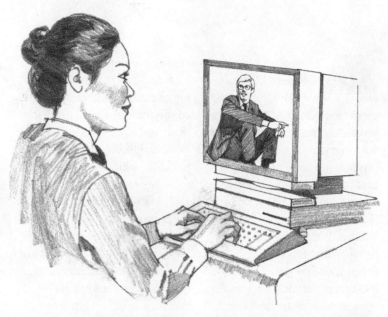

Whether you work in the office or at home on a personal computer, you must provide your own protection. The essential ergonomic question—how does it feel to work with this machine and its peripherals all day?—has become the single most important consideration when purchasing a computer. Think first about the way the computer itself *feels*, then deal with the peripherals.

How Easy Is It to Use?

Computer ads, like automobile ads, emphasize speed, power and performance while ignoring the fact that human beings must find a way to operate the machine. Buy the wrong machine and you will find yourself longing for the good old electric typewriter. As system crashes, software failures and printer incompatibilities paralyze your office for hours (even days), you will dream about tossing the computer out the window and watching it shatter on the street below.

Forget about Power and Speed

First, ask simply, how hard is the machine to use? (In computerese: how friendly is the user interface?) Artificial intelligence research has yielded computers that are beginning to be intuitive; rather than type a string of arcane commands, you simply point to an item on the screen. A friendly user interface could make the difference between success or frustration in your office. You can't mistake the feel of an ergonomic interface; it allows the beginner to feel confident, the casual user to get up to speed quickly and the experienced user to access the full power of a computer efficiently.

An intuitive icon

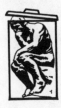

User Interface: How to Get Started

	Good	Bad
Stuck?	On-screen help menus. An 800 help number with a knowledgeable staff	Look it up in a huge manual written by programmers. Call the manufacturer at your expense
Advanced user?	Speed up with short cuts	Only one method
Beginner?	Controls are intuitive	System presents an ocean of unfamiliar symbols and commands
Expanding?	Standard approaches to all programs	Different commands for each program
Printing?	What you see on the screen is identical to what you get from the printer	A surprise each time

Laptop and Notebook Computers

At first glance the diminutive laptop or notebook computer seems to be an ideal solution for people who want a machine that does everything. It's light, thin, compact, portable and has a small footprint. Since the screen doesn't use a cathode ray tube (CRT), virtually no radiation is emitted. But whether or not a laptop will be ergonomic for you depends on how you plan to use it. Some of the most attractive features have distinct ergonomic drawbacks.

Small LCD screens become difficult to read during long sessions. Active matrix screens provide better resolution but at a considerably higher cost. The cramped keyboard, generally attached to the screen, harkens back to the first one-piece desktop computers whose awkward configurations forced users to bend and squint while they worked. Finally, a fixed position trackball, while handy for short sessions, reduces flexibility.

Think of a laptop as a traveling computer and you will appreciate its convenience. However, if you also plan to use it as your main machine, consider adding a larger CRT screen, a detached ergonomic keyboard and a separate pointing device such as a mouse or trackball, accessories that are easily disconnected for travel.

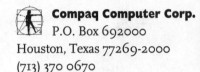

Compaq Computer Corp.
P.O. Box 692000
Houston, Texas 77269-2000
(713) 370 0670

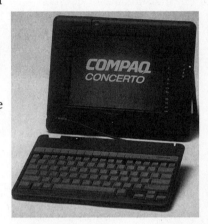

A notebook computer with a detachable keyboard.

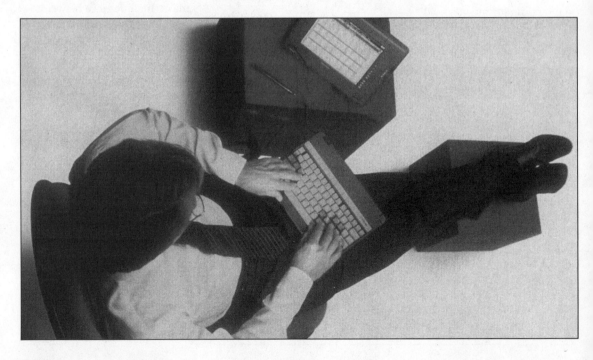

Keyboards

Early typewriters relied on a forest of clattering metal spokes, with tiny characters fastened to the ends, to get a letter from keyboard to paper. Hitting a key hard enough activated a complex network of cams and gears that finally propelled a single spoke forward. If everything worked, the character on the spoke top was forced against a narrow fabric ribbon and finally

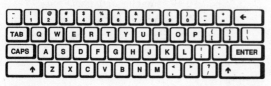

Standard QWERTY layout

imprinted on paper. However, with so many intricately linked, moving parts, everything didn't always work.

A fast typist could easily outpace the flailing spokes, bringing on the massive key jams that were eventually accepted as a necessary evil. So the typewriter, which began life as a labor-saving device, began to create new jobs for writers. Spokes had to be untangled and straightened, ribbons adjusted, tiny pieces of type cleaned, while inside the machine a vast

network of gears and levers needed regular oiling and fine tuning. The faster a person typed, the more often some mysterious part failed; users either spent more time typing or more time on maintenance.

Given the limited technology of the time, the most ergonomic solution seemed to be an uneasy compromise between typists and their balky machines. When manufacturers realized that the only way to save typewriters was to slow down typists, the QWERTY keyboard, named after

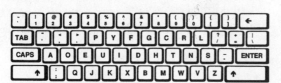

Two-handed Dvorak layout

the row of letters on the top left-hand side, was born. Several of the most common letters had to be typed by the pinkie. It was one of the *slowest possible* keyboard layouts.

Keytime
4516 N.E. 54th Street
Seattle, Washington 98105
(206) 524 2238

Carpal Tunnel Syndrome

Once the workplace becomes an assembly line, machines set the pace and people follow. When mechanization and automation lightened the workload the *pace* of work accelerated. Suddenly going to work meant typing and dialing furiously and repeating little jobs with the fingers instead of doing a few big jobs with the legs and back. Stresses that were once borne by the body's largest muscles were now concentrated on some of the smallest—in the hands.

Pain and Typing

You don't usually think of the hands as a source of great physical pain. To use your hands in an office usually means to type, telephone or write, jobs that require little muscle power.

Nonetheless, the muscles of the hands can wear as surely as the muscles of the back, and the results can be just as devastating. An excruciatingly painful variety of repetitive motion syndrome, caused by cumulative overuse of the hands, afflicts thousands of typists. You pay the penalty for poor typing ergonomics every waking hour.

It doesn't take an evil organization or an ambitious office manager to create this problem. The computer is such an efficient, tireless tool that people *want* to work hard at it. But where do they stop? Overeager young newspaper reporters have been quite literally paralyzed by too much typing.

Uninformed co-workers blame the victim—"don't tell

Cumulative trauma pain begins in the shaded areas.

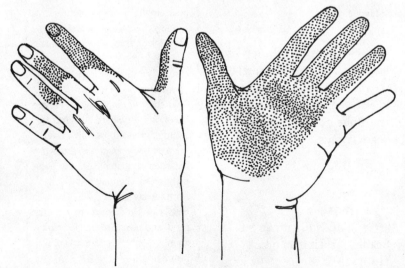

SOURCE: *Cumulative Trauma Disorders: A Manual for Musculoskeletal Diseases of the Upper Limbs,* VERN PUTZ-ANDERSON, Taylor and Francis, Philadelphia, 1990.

Symptoms of CTS

Tingling

At first CTS is insidious: initially you feel a painful tingling in one or both hands at night, perhaps enough to wake you after a few hours of sleep. Then, they start tingling and hurting in the daytime. Your fingers feel swollen: it becomes difficult to tell hot from cold or to squeeze things.

Finger Pain

You begin to notice a nagging pain in the first three fingers and at the base of the thumb.

Weak Hands

In advanced cases the muscle at the base of the thumb actually atrophies. The hands look dry and shiny from lack of sweat, and they feel clumsy and weak.

me you can't type"—while victims too easily blame other factors such as arthritis or aging.

However, the pain caused by cumulative trauma disorder comes from an accumulation of little injuries called *microtraumas,* which begs for ergonomic solutions.

Inside the Hands

The fingers are controlled by a bundle of flexor tendons that connect to the muscles in the forearm. These tendons share a tight sheath of ligaments with the median nerve. The whole bundle must squeeze through a narrow tunnel at the wrist where the carpal bones meet the hand. If the hands (or nearby muscles in the arms) are constantly used improperly, the tendons become inflamed, putting direct pressure on the median nerve.

Are You at Risk?

Repetitive motion syndrome (carpal tunnel syndrome, or CTS, being only one kind) isn't limited to the office. Athletes who must repeat the same arm movement know the problem as tennis (or golfer's) elbow.

Office workers suffer whenever the same job is repeated too many times. The keyboard operator and typist share similar complaints with the telephone operator (leaning on the elbow against a hard desk causes irritation of the ulnar nerve, which leads to numbness and pain in the little finger). The newest complaints, *mousing elbow* and *space invaders wrist*, caused by too many video games, follow the familiar pattern that typists know so well.

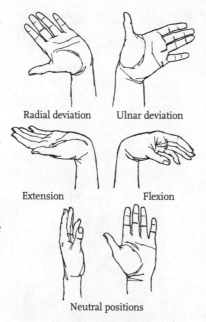

Radial deviation   Ulnar deviation

Extension   Flexion

Neutral positions

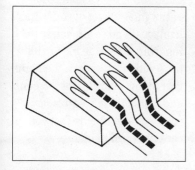

It takes more effort to complete a task with a bent wrist than with the wrist in a neutral position.

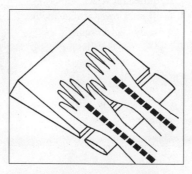

Combining a low-profile keyboard with a soft wristpad keeps your wrists in a neutral position.

Flirting with CTS

You risk CTS if you are:

Gripping, twisting, reaching or moving repeatedly without rest or sufficient recovery time and without change.

Extending your wrist both downward and upward.

Permitting a computer to set the pace.

Repeating motions that put your hand, wrist or elbow in contact with sharp or hard edges.

Working in low temperatures.

Attempting to work in an awkward, fixed or constrained posture.

The Pain of CTS

What causes your pain:

Hands and wrists: A sharp-edged desk, a high-lipped keyboard, or other input tools such as mice, trackballs and graphics tablets amplify stresses.

Shoulder and neck: No support for the arms puts an extra strain on upper body muscles.

Arms and hands: Attempting to support your elbows on a hard surface or armrest (or simply leaning on a hard desk) can lead to a pinched ulnar nerve.

Hazardous Jobs

Computer users, cooks, carpenters, photographers and meat packers have one thing in common: they all do work with repetitive, small hand movements that put them at risk for carpal tunnel syndrome.

CTS affects women more often than men. Women are at greatest risk during pregnancy and other conditions in which the hands are likely to swell.

Repetitive Tasks

You're at risk if your job requires:
  data entry
  record keeping
  word processing
  mail order processing
  telephone directory
    assistance

Legislation

Legislation and guidelines have been enacted in Sweden, Australia and the United States. Both Sweden and Australia have tried to allow workers enough control over their work posture and movements to avoid injury. The U.S. guidelines focus on prevention through tool, job and task design, as well as training.

Help for CTS Sufferers

The antidote to CTS is a combination of ergonomic design and adequate rest. Simply vary-

Basic Ergonomics

Start by reevaluating the items you use while typing:

Chair
  Adjustable arm supports (with no loss of lumbar support) made from padded non-slip material

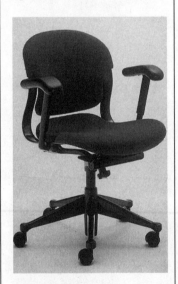

Desk
  Softly rounded edge and the right height, which should keep your lower arm at about a ninety-degree angle to the upper arm while typing

Keyboard
  Top quality, detached, low profile with low, rounded wrist support

ing your job, stretching and taking more breaks will make a difference. If you're already suffering from CTS, you probably need therapy and medical intervention. In order to return to work, you may have to put ergonomics first and modify the way your job is done.

Left untreated, CTS can lead to significant and lasting disability. If mild symptoms have been present for less than two months, conservative treatment that restricts motion with a splint, coupled with anti-inflammatory drugs, may cure the problem over time. It takes weeks and often months for medical therapy to be successful. Cases with severe symptoms may require surgery.

To heal properly, the stresses *causing* CTS must be removed. Take it slow if you're returning from an injury or starting on a job. Don't expect a single change to make much difference; you must evaluate the entire inner circle of your office habitat. If you're already suffering from CTS or working full time with a computer, the items that follow—keyboards, screens and workstations—provide ergonomic solutions that you cannot afford to ignore.

Hand Tools

It shouldn't come as a surprise that we have developed computer keyboards capable of destroying our hands. Abusive hand tools have been with us for centuries.

The hand is so flexible that we expect it to work in virtually any position. If it aches, we treat the symptoms and go on working with the offending tool. During intensive typing, however, we've had to recognize that forcing the wrist joint into an awkward position for hours on end is a sure recipe for distressing pain. Typing becomes even more difficult if we routinely abuse our hands during other tasks.

Don't wait for the pain to begin. If you have trouble typing on "standard" keyboards you will experience difficulties with other badly designed hand tools. Most clumsy, conventional tools have elegant ergonomic counterparts that spare your hands and make typing, when you return to it, less stressful.

You feel the difference the moment you begin working with an ergonomic tool.

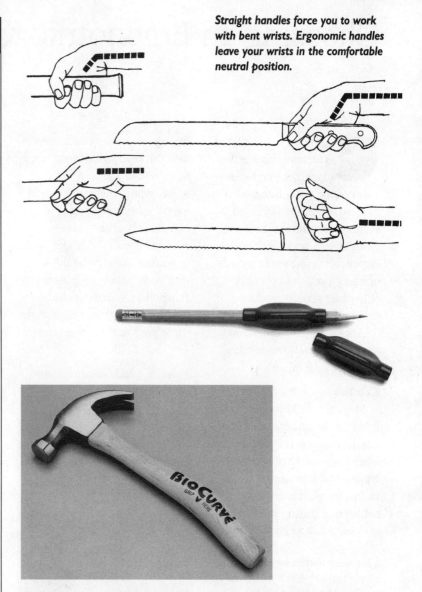

Straight handles force you to work with bent wrists. Ergonomic handles leave your wrists in the comfortable neutral position.

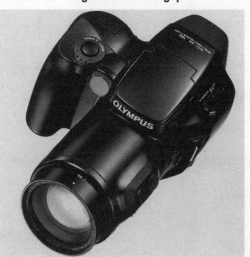

Ergonomic camera grip

North Coast Medical
187 Stauffer Boulevard
San Jose, California 95125-1042
(800) 821 9319

Olympus Corporation
145 Crossways Park
Woodbury, New York 11797-2087
(516) 364 3000

Choosing an Ergonomic Keyboard

Compared to the host of expensive, high-tech machines that have crowded their way into the modern office, the keyboard seems small and insignificant. Nevertheless, good keyboard ergonomics can save hundreds of hours a year and prevent potentially serious medical problems.

Ask these questions when you choose an ergonomic keyboard for your office:

Can You Move It ?

Moving your keyboard away from the computer allows you, not the computer, to decide where you will sit or stand while typing. Mobility almost always makes for good ergonomics. At some point during the day you may want to lean back, put your

A keyboard that combines a wrist support with a split center to correct for ulnar deviation

feet up on the desk and type with the keyboard in your lap. Not too long ago your high school typing instructor would have flunked you for that maneuver, but she was more concerned with the health of the typewriter than the health of your body. Most computers with attached keyboards, including the most desirable laptops, have some provision for plugging in

If your chair lacks adjustable arms, attach them to your desk.

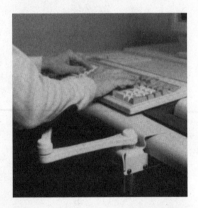

an external one. Doing so will change your whole day. Be sure the cord is long enough for you to type comfortably with the keyboard in your lap.

Can You Rest Your Wrists on the Desk While Typing?

Fatigue, which affects the whole upper body, especially the neck and shoulders, begins the moment you start typing with your wrists in the air. Try it for a moment; you will instantly feel the difference in the muscles of your fingers and arms and then, moments later, across the neck and shoulders. It doesn't take long for poor keyboard ergonomics to create serious aches and pains.

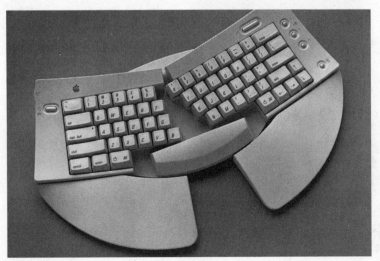

AliMed
297 High Street
Dedham, Massachusetts 02026
(800) 225 2610

Apple Computer, Inc.
20525 Mariani Avenue
Cupertino, California 95014

The ergonomic solution—a comfortably sloped keyboard with a soft, low front lip—permits you to rest your wrists on the desktop while supporting the upper arms. As you type you can see the keys without bending forward. Older high-lipped keyboards become more comfortable when you add a sloped wedge in front. The most ergonomic keyboards are supported by a low rubber bumper that also provides a cushioned support for the wrists.

Think of the keyboard, the workstation (tabletop) and the chair as an interconnected system for supporting your arms, wrists and back. If you must lean forward to type, you're likely to get a backache. The same thing will happen if your armrests are too long. Without a place to rest the arms, upper back and shoulders might become tired from bearing the weight of your arms all day. The edge of the table and that of the keyboard need to be softly rounded, preventing damage to your wrists as they move across these surfaces. Hard and narrow armrests can add to the problems by putting pressure on the ulnar nerve in the elbow.

Can You Feel the Keys Making Contact while You Type?

Liberated from the din of manual typewriters, some computer manufacturers produced machines with completely silent

keyboards. This "breakthrough" turned out to be bad ergonomics simply because most typists prefer an auditory cue in addition to the purely tactile each time a letter is typed. Avoid keyboards with overly mushy keys that fail to provide the crucial tactile and auditory feedback necessary for fast typing.

Can You Type Quickly without Sipping Off the Keys?

Flat key caps, which make it impossible to stop your fingers from slipping and sliding as you work, will reduce the fastest touch typist to a hunt-and-peck crawl. Sculpted keys that are fitted to the pads of your fingers provide a simple ergonomic solution. Raised dots on the D and K or, occasionally, the F and J keys help a touch typist work without studying the keyboard.

Desktop Layout: What Works and What Doesn't

There are two schools of thought—the purist demands an uncluttered, basic keyboard with an absolute minimum of function keys. Traditional, memory-taxing function keys are replaced by a pointing device, such as a mouse, which can be used to select options from an array of intuitive symbols on pull-down menus. The traditionalist argues that reaching for a mouse slows down the commonly used commands, all of which can be easily executed from the keyboard with special keys. Decide for yourself—what's ergonomic for one typist might not be so for another. Testing your software on various keyboards (there are dozens for all the popular computers) helps to determine the ideal layout. Since keyboards are generally not bundled with a computer, you need not automatically settle for the one that's made by the manufacturer of your machine.

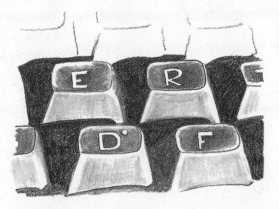

Mice, Trackballs and Tablets

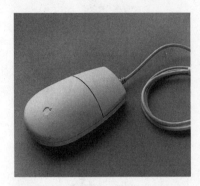

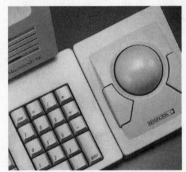

Since typing is a repetitive chore, even the best keyboard represents an ergonomic compromise. In the future, people will talk directly to their computers; all the major computer manufacturers are working on speech-augmented keyboards.

Meanwhile, a host of clever new input devices have already arrived. A numeric keypad turns the keyboard into a calculator.

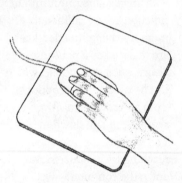

The mouse makes pointing easier, but demands valuable desk space. A mouse pad corrects the mouse's tendency to slip on hard surfaces. The trackball duplicates most mouse capabilities while remaining in one spot.

Apple Computer, Inc.
20525 Mariani Avenue
Cupertino, California 95014

Pointing Device Ergonomics

Keyboard connections

Devices that can be attached to the sides of a keyboard, rather than the computer itself, are much more flexible. If you're left-handed, choose a system that permits input devices to be attached on the left side of the keyboard.

Tool design

Like the standard keyboard, input tools should have a sloping profile with soft edges and good tactile (even auditory) feedback. Avoid a shiny mouse. Every bit of glare protection helps.

Specialized pointing devices like the joystick, used primarily for games, and the graphics tablet, which is a drawing tool, improve on the keyboard. Other keyboard alternatives have created, rather than solved, ergonomic problems. Commands displayed on a *touch screen* require users to press their fingertips against the surface of the CRT itself, a punishing action on a vertical surface. Touch screens and displays that accept handwriting work better on screens that emulate pads of paper. You will write more comfortably by hand on a screen that lies flat on your desk.

Kensington
2855 Campus Drive
San Mateo, California 94403
(800) 535 4242

Screens

The lowly computer screen, also known as the monitor, CRT or video display terminal (VDT), may cause more aches and pains per square inch than any labor-saving device ever invented.

If you've come to a computer from a typewriter, you're probably accustomed to working with ordinary black type on white paper in a brightly lighted room, perhaps with a window near the desk. But now, suddenly, the simple act of reading your own writing takes on ominous new dimensions. Switching on the computer, you're confronted with rows of uncertain luminous characters that pulsate slowly against a black background. Numbers roll and jitter; strange reflections distract you. You then must squint, crane your neck and turn up the brightness control until rows of incandescent green characters scroll merrily across the downtown skyline.

The eyes usually go first, blurring, then burning at odd hours. Soon chronic neck pain begins, followed by terrifying lower-back spasms. Welcome to the computer revolution. Press *print*, think of the time you've just saved and gulp a couple of aspirin.

But wait! The green screen is almost history, flickering displays can be controlled and glare eliminated. Ergonomic alternatives to yesterday's stress-inducing screen are emerging every day. In fact, you may be surprised at just how much control you actually have over stress-inducing video terminals.

For starters, consider the major ergonomic advantages in choosing the correct size and color for your screen. Flicker, glare and uncomfortable posture are no longer part of the daily price you must pay.

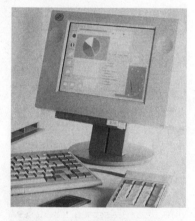

A flat screen that swivels, pivots and has a small footprint

Eliminate them and you will free yourself from dozens of aches and pains that torture computer users needlessly.

If you don't already have a computer, you're likely to get one soon. Millions of workers already use CRTs. As their ranks grow daily, so do their health complaints. The wrong screen can cause all kinds of health problems, but computer operators also require ergonomic chairs, desks and illumination. Before you blame your CRT, look carefully at your whole habitat. The following information is for readers who hurt after the first week at a new computer.

You suffer because you fall into working habits with a CRT that you would never tolerate with a typewriter or any other machine. That's why screen ergonomics must focus on a single concern, which becomes far more important than the computer's memory, speed or software: the computer is tireless and you are not. Sure, you're saving plenty of time, but at what cost to your health?

Even though you're sitting on a hard wooden stool under banks of glaring lights, a computer manages to provide instantaneous feedback, keeping you riveted to the screen hour after hour. Clerical jobs that once required getting up frequently—to file, put new paper in the typewriter, look up words in a dictionary—have become utterly sedentary. Without exercise, stress levels climb, and that's only the beginning.

IBM
133 Westchester Avenue
White Plains, New York 10604
(800) 772 2227

Hidden Stress and Solutions

The computer is still so new that many users will endure glare all day without realizing it.

Are You Squinting as You Use Your Computer?

Can you see an image of yourself in the screen?

Can you see an image of a light source in the screen?

Are portions of the screen difficult to see?

If the answer to any of the above questions is *yes,* you are probably struggling with glare. Light from windows, even reflected natural light, almost always causes problems. Even when you perceive little discomfort, say, from a window in your peripheral view, the long-term effect will be eye irritation.

Never think about glare as an isolated problem reserved for your computer screen. Yes, the screen certainly does pick up

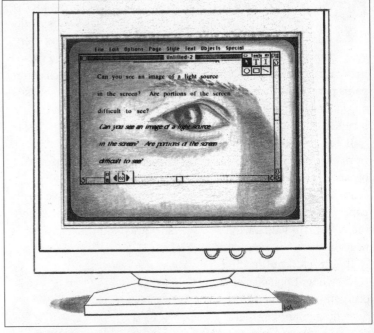

reflected light, but the most effective way to control it involves rethinking the illumination patterns in your office. First, locate the sources of visible screen glare: a window behind your desk, a lamp aimed directly at the screen. Then, see

if you can reposition your computer so that no visible light falls on it. Failing that, cover the windows with an opaque shade that can be lowered when the sun shines. Old-style, fluorescent lighting that flickers overhead is universally disliked by computer workers; *full spectrum* fluorescents are the preferred choices, (see p. 132). Switching to narrow focus task lamps will allow you to illuminate your desk without including your screen.

Luxo Lamp Company
36 Midland Avenue
Port Chester, New York 10573
(914) 937 4433

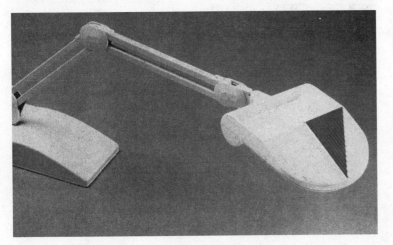

Ambient Lights

Avoid extremely bright rooms for computer work. You need less than half as much ambient light for computing than for general office work. Lowering the ambient light diminishes the contrast between the screen and your surroundings and thus immediately reduces reflections and glare. Add dimmers on all switches. If you're looking for a fast, temporary solution, simply disconnect selected overhead lights. Most offices have too much ambient light.

Task lights

Since nearly everyone needs to do traditional kinds of office work, think about ways to complement the lowered ambient light with task lights (see p. 133). Each one should be adjustable, ideally both in direction and intensity. The classic gooseneck lamp is a good inexpensive choice.

Windows

Most computers are installed in an existing office environment. If you have just one window, put the computer screen on a desk placed at a ninety-degree angle to the window. Whatever glare you do pick up will be on the peripheral side of one eye. This setup also prevents reflections in the screen and eliminates the terrible glare problems you encounter when facing a window or the brightly lighted wall opposite one. Any peripheral glare can easily be reduced by a blind on the window.

A fifteen-inch screen that pivots to display a vertical or horizontal page

Tinted Eyeglasses

Lightly tinted eyeglasses can help cut screen glare even further. Light gray, brown and pink tints can be combined with reading lenses, if necessary, to keep both written copy and screen information clear. Investigate tinted "computer glasses" with your optometrist.

Contrast

The ergonomic issue in illuminating the office is determining how much contrast will work for you. If you do detail work in a room that requires some artificial lighting, a sunlit window will interfere with your concentration every time you

Radius Inc.
1710 Fortune Drive
San Jose, California 95131
(408) 434 1010

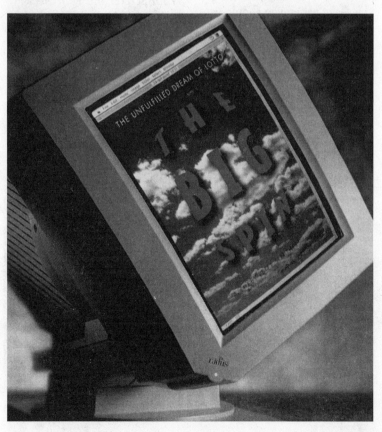

glance up. The window becomes intolerable if it's directly opposite your computer screen.

Flicker

The image that you actually see on your traditional CRT monitor is retransmitted or refreshed (redrawn) many times each second. If the refresh rate is too slow the screen will flicker noticeably. Since faster refresh rates required faster computers, the first generation of monitors featured slow screens that did nothing to control flicker. Thanks to faster computer chips, screen speed is no longer a significant issue; there's simply no excuse anymore for a flickering display.

Screen Size

Since large screens are so expensive and bulky, most com-

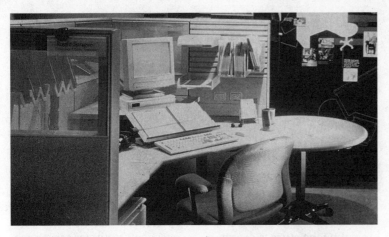

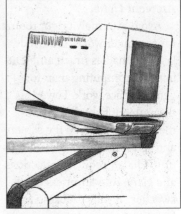

puter users make do with small ones. Apart from the reduced footprint, there are no good reasons to use small screens. Inexpensive larger screens (and eventually flat ones with minimal footprints) will someday be available. For now, the ergonomic question remains: who really needs a large screen? A simple ergonomic rule applies here: if you work with large pieces of paper, you should use a large screen.

Footprint

Think about fitting a twenty-inch television set onto your desk—how much space would be left for you? Big monitors hog vast chunks of desk space. Yes, you may need a new monitor, but if you can't manage a new desk you may simply create new ergonomic problems by solving the old ones. An adjustable arm permits you to keep the desk you now have by moving the monitor to a floating platform above your desktop. This zero-footprint solution preserves your desk space. Simply move the monitor out of the way when you're not using it.

Your Screen and Your Neck

The head is a very heavy object that must be supported by the neck and shoulders all day long. Don't create extra work for your body. Position your screen so you can view it at an angle just slightly lower than straight ahead. Since people sit at differing heights, a computer screen should be adjustable in order to get a comfortable viewing angle. Some computers come with a "foot" or sometimes an arm that allows for tilting, swiveling, raising and lowering the screen. Specialized computer desks help position the screen. A less expensive solution is to simply prop the CRT on a homemade wedge to create a decent viewing angle, but if more than one person uses the computer an adjustable CRT becomes essential.

AliMed
297 High Street
Dedham, Massachusetts 02026
(800) 225 2610

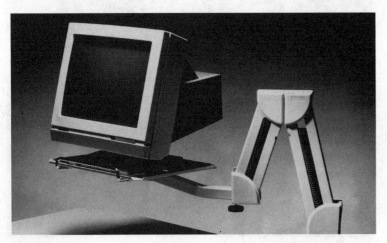

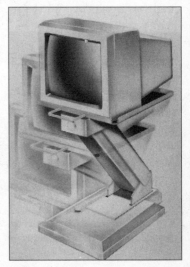

Screens and Color

Your eyes actually see certain colors far more precisely than others. While yellow focuses squarely on the retina, red, blue and green are concentrated on either side. You may not notice it right away, but blue or green text will always appear slightly blurred. Red and violet not only focus poorly but are more difficult to see than other colors.

Monochrome Screens

Avoid green characters on a black background whenever possible. This combination can produce a kind of visual pollution including an irritating pink afterimage, known as the McCullogh Effect.

The standard for office computers should be black text on a whitish background. Since we're all familiar with black text on white paper (we usually print that way) this is an obvious ergonomic choice. However, black text on an amber background, favored in parts of Europe, can be more restful for the eyes.

Color Screens

When color was confined to scientific applications and games, the main problem was how to print things. This has been changing rapidly over the last couple of years as high-quality color printers have plummeted in price. Color monitors and color output will open

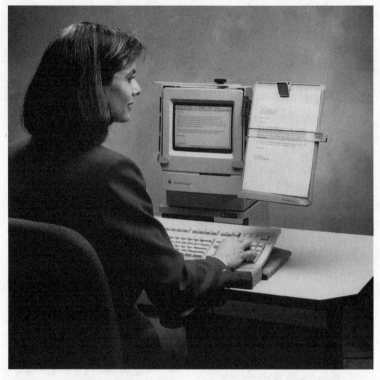

A copy stand brings reading material up to the same height and angle as your screen, reducing strain on your neck and shoulders.

up uncharted territory for the office computer user.

However, it will still be important to be able to convey information with elements *other* than color. (Bear in mind that nearly 10 percent of all men and .5 percent of all women have some degree of color blindness.) Mixing black outlining with your color will highlight important items. Color combinations that are difficult to see on the screen will remain difficult when printed. Blue text

on a red background might seem refreshing after all those hours spent looking at black characters, but ultimately your audience will struggle to read it.

North Coast Medical, Inc.
187 Stauffer Boulevard
San Jose, California 95125-1042
(800) 821 9319

Your Screen and Your Eyes

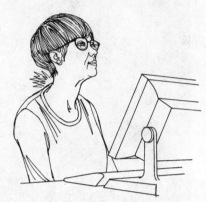

How important is CRT ergonomics? Drop a computer into a work situation with no ergonomic preparation and by the end of the first week you're likely to hear the familiar refrain: "My eyes hurt and I'm always tired."

The eyes are often the first part of the body to register fatigue, even when the cause may be postural. The symptoms include itching, burning, aching, soreness and watering. Once fatigue sets in, vision blurs.

All closely detailed clerical work causes eye strain. The more tedious and poorly paid the work (such as intensive data processing with poor copy), the more complaints. Of course, eye problems can be caused by other ergonomic factors (see pp. 127–33), but poor CRT ergonomics will make a difficult situation intolerable.

Backaches and Bifocals

More than half of full-time computer users complain of back and shoulder problems. Women tend to have upper-back pain while men complain of lower-back pain. The upper-back pain is often associated with head and neck aches, another common complaint. Here again, look at the whole habitat, especially the chair. Simply changing your eyeglass-es may relieve a host of mysterious aches and pains.

Half glasses (for reading) and bifocals are designed to be used with the reading material resting on a tabletop. When the reader's head is bent slightly toward a desktop, the eyes can peer over the top of the glasses (or through the upper half of the bifocals) at more distant objects. This system, which has worked well for the past two hundred years, precipitates an ergonomic crisis for computer users. Attempting to read a vertical display with bifocals means forcing your entire head into a permanent backward tilt. Yes, you can do it, but within hours aches and pains blossom in the neck and shoulders.

You'll probably need an extra pair of glasses for computer work—a small price to pay for a relaxed body. But first, try dispensing with your eyeglasses altogether. Push the screen back on the desktop and (if your computer permits) use a larger screen font for your work. If you still need help reading the screen, get a pair of full reading glasses to use for computer work.

CRT Eye Care

Do:
    Use a glare filter
    Adjust intensity
    Adjust height
    Adjust tilt
    Adjust angle
    Lower ambient light
    Eye exercises

Don't:
    Wear bifocals or half-glasses
    Stare into a window or bright wall
    Wear contacts (if your eyes bother you)
    Ignore pain in your eyes

Eye Care

CRT work is visually demanding. When was the last time you checked your eyeglass prescription?

If you wear contact lenses, itchiness, dryness and discomfort may be caused by the dry air and static electricity that surround most CRTs. Use a static-electricity shield (see p. 167). Wear regular glasses.

You must schedule breaks to give your eyes a rest. When taking a break, avoid close eye work like reading or knitting. Instead allow your eyes to relax by looking out the window, taking a walk or even just engaging in conversation.

Take a walking meeting; exercise isn't the only benefit. Happily, the most restful position for the eyes is long-distance seeing.

Focusing Exercises
Repeat several times.

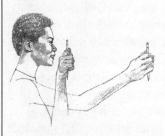

1. Medium-distance gazing. Follow the pencil with your eyes while you move it in and out slowly.

2. Long-distance gazing. Start by repeating medium-distance gazing. When your hand gets furthest away from your face let your eyes focus on a distant object.

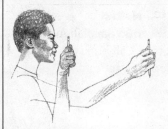

Palming
Repeat several times.

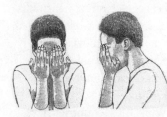

Cup your hands over your eyes, and hold them in place for awhile. Breathe deeply, visualize something pleasant and restful. Palming brings instant rest to the eyes. Repeat it after each set of eye exercises.

Peripheral Vision Exercises
Repeat several times.

One eye at a time. Hold a pencil in your hand and move it slowly as far to the side as you can see. Follow the pencil with your eye while keeping your head straight.

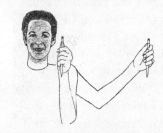

2. Both eyes at once. Look at both pencils while you move them out to both sides simultaneously.

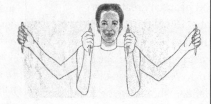

Radiation: Are You Being Zapped?

Serious research on CRT radiation now focuses on components inside the computer monitor that produce radiation at *very low frequencies* (VLF) and *extremely low frequencies* (ELF) and generate an insidious, weak electromagnetic field. CRTs are painted from within by a fast-moving electron beam that emits pulses of electrical energy. A powerful static electrical field is also created in front of the monitor, causing dust and airborne contaminants to cling to your face. (The same static field attracts dust to your television screen.) The side effects of this field alone could be a major cause of CRT health complaints. Happily, you can easily intercept static electricity. More on that in a moment.

The effects of electromagnetic radiation are not nearly as well understood. In fact, many household appliances (electric blankets, power tools, vacuum cleaners, hair dryers and waterbed heaters) create more intense low-frequency electromagnetic fields than CRTs whenever they are operated. If we don't shield ourselves from a blender, should we be afraid of a computer?

Scientists once held that unless low-frequency electromagnetic radiation was intense enough to transmit heat, there was nothing to worry about. This assumption has now been questioned by consumer groups with concerns about the effects of low-frequency radiation on human reproduction.[1]

In 1985 the World Heath Organization (WHO) declared that CRT emissions cannot be regarded as hazardous and that available data does not support claims of links between CRT use and reproductive harm. At the same time the WHO acknowledged that damaging effects of electromagnetic radiation cannot be completely ruled out. Since then, however, evidence of the possible harmful effects of radiation has been mounting.

While most countries have not established a safe standard of exposure to electromagnetic radiation, the Swedish government took a stronger stand,

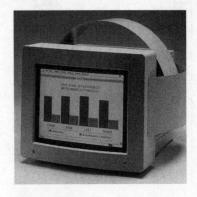

Clip-on radiation shield

insisting that CRT manufacturers eliminate electrostatic fields and substantially reduce low-frequency electromagnetic radiation in all units sold within the country.

No conclusive evidence, as yet, indicates that CRTs produce dangerous radiation. Yet the preliminary studies are worrisome enough for *Consumer Reports* to conclude that "computers have come under suspicion because of the electromagnetic fields they create."[2] We suggest you stay informed.

NoRad
1160 Sandhill Avenue
Carson, California 90746
(800) 262 3260

Skin Rashes

Skin rashes, reported in Scandinavia, where CRT health studies have been taken seriously for years, may be caused by hot dry air generated by computers and their peripherals. Dry air also amplifies a potentially more serious problem: the strong static electrical charge put out by all CRTs causes dust and allergens to stick to your face. A static shield (p. 167) and humidifier will protect your skin.

1. "The Magnetic Field Menace," by Paul Brodeur, *Macworld* magazine, July 1990.

2. "Electromagnetic Fields," *Consumer Reports*, May 1994, p. 358.

How to Protect Yourself

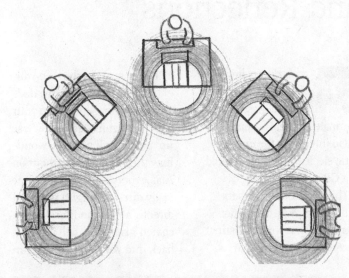

CRT seating arrangement

Low-emission monitors which reduce the insidious low-end electromagnetic field are finally becoming available here in the United States (IBM and Apple have supplied them for years in Sweden). Laptop computers using liquid crystal display (the same technology used in calculators and watches) generate no electromagnetic radiation. However, most of these displays are still inferior to the CRT and too difficult to read for full-time use. Happily, flat-screen technology is moving fast; radiation-free high-quality flat displays will eventually replace the CRT.

Meanwhile, to be on the safe side, set up your seating arrangements so people are not sitting directly behind somebody else's CRT. Electromagnetic radiation is generated by the flyback transformer that rests against the rear of the monitor. Effective protection for everyone in an office requires either shielding the sides plus the back and front of each CRT or maintaining a reasonable distance. The weak field, which diminishes sharply at fifteen inches, is virtually unmeasurable at thirty inches.

For the Pregnant User

Some electromagnetic-field studies indicate the possibility of harmful effects to mice and chicken embryos. While this research continues, governments, labor unions, manufacturers and users struggle with the implications for pregnant women.

If you're pregnant and work with a computer, don't focus solely on the radiation question. First, do a complete ergonomic evaluation of your workstation including the chair, desk, climate control, keyboard, vision and positioning of the computer screen. Install a screen filter that will eliminate static electricity. Then, consider the monitor itself.

Many CRTs sold in the United States still do not intercept the controversial low-frequency electromagnetic field. Choose one that guarantees that it meets the Swedish standards for radiation (sometimes designated by the symbol MPR-2). If you have an older machine, simply sitting back an arm's length from your monitor will put you safely outside the field. If you prefer to sit close to your CRT or if you work in a crowded office, consider an external clip-on magnetic radiation shield.

"We cannot sit idly waiting for the [radiation] research findings to come through. If we really mean what we say about taking people's apprehensions seriously, we must also be prepared to take unconfirmed but suspected risks into account. . . . Although there is no evidence today of this radiation having any biological effects, there is no reason for burdening the occupational environment with factors that can be eliminated."[1] Based on this conclusion, the Swedish civil service and numerous public and private entities made agreements that provide for the transfer of pregnant women to non-CRT work without loss of pay or seniority.

1. Swedish Labor Minister Anna Greta Lejon, opening address at the Work with Display Units conference, Stockholm 1986.

Eliminating CRT Glare and Reflections

A polarized filter with transparent, metal coated glass virtually eliminates glare. If grounded, it also intercepts the entire static electrical field generated by a CRT.

The effect on CRT users couldn't be more dramatic; characters that were indistinct are suddenly crystal clear.

If you want to show co-workers what ergonomics can do, add one of these filters to your CRT. Five minutes after it's set up, people will begin to wonder how they managed without one. Alas, when a bright light (especially direct sunlight) is aimed directly at the monitor, the coated-glass filter will reflect it back into your eyes. If you can-

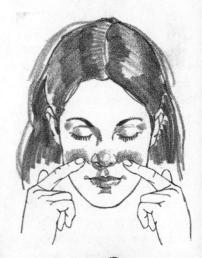

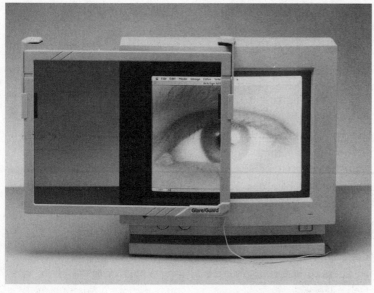

Polarized screen

 OCLI
Santa Rosa, California 95497
(707) 545 6440

not redirect the light source, consider a metallic mesh filter, an ergonomic solution that reduces reflections as well as glare.

The mesh does cause minor degradation of the visual image, but most people who work in sunlit rooms will agree that the trade-off is worth it.

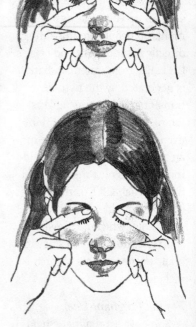

Putting pressure on the sinuses helps to relieve CRT-generated eye fatigue.

Printing Your Work

Printer advertising almost always emphasizes only two features: speed, measured in pages per minute (or characters per second on the older dot matrix printers) and the quality of the type and graphics. However, the difference between printers that are capable of, say, three and four pages per minute is far less important than their respective paper-handling capabilities. A difficult printer will generate horrifying paper delays that instantly reduce output to zero pages per minute, a rate it will maintain until you manage to get paper to flow or feed properly through the machine. In printers, nothing matters more

Printer Ergonomics

Ask these questions about the printer's paper-handling capabilities:

Does it work with ordinary paper?

Is it easy to load?

How difficult is it to change from draft-quality paper to correspondence quality?

Does it print envelopes, and if so, how difficult are they to load?

Does paper slip out of alignment during printing?

Will it accept single sheets of your letterhead paper?

How difficult is it to fix a paper jam?

than efficient paper handling.

Output Quality

Once you're satisfied with a printer's paper handling, move on to other ergonomic considerations. First, evaluate a printed page on good-quality paper. Ignore manufacturers' claims regarding *letter-quality* text, a dated term that refers to a printer's ability to emulate the output of an IBM Selectric typewriter. This is rather like selecting a car for its ability to ride like a horse. Many inexpensive printers can now emulate the quality of commercial printing presses, producing near-book-quality output with a host of graphic abilities that no typewriter can approach.

Compatibility

Your printer must be fully compatible with the software you intend to use. Perhaps you need scientific notation, graphic symbols or foreign language characters. Once the necessary software has been selected, the vital ergonomic question becomes, how closely does what you see on the screen of your computer resemble what you actually get from the printer? This ergonomic requirement is so important that it has its own acronym among computer users: WYSIWYG, what you see is what you get.

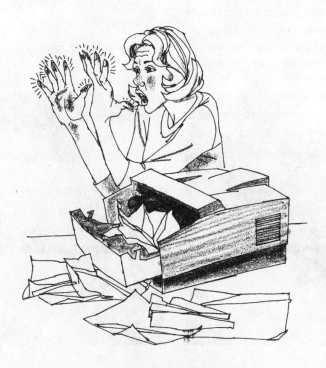

Choosing a Printer

Among the first questions you'll want to ask about the printer are, how much space does it require and where are you going to put it? Then, where will your printed work emerge from the printer? On dot matrix printers, lengthy documents may require floor space to create a folded stack. Add together the necessary printer space and floor space to avoid underestimating the amount of room your printer will actually need. To protect your precious desk space, consider a separate table for your printer.

Cartridges

Printers use ink or ribbon cartridges that must be easy to change and readily available in your area. Don't let your entire office grind to a halt while you hunt for a nonstandard cartridge.

Noise

The buzz-saw whine of a noisy dot matrix printer (fortunately, these are being replaced by quieter mechanisms) will penetrate every corner of your office and get on your nerves. Specially designed sound boxes are clumsy to work with but virtually a necessity with these machines. A sound-absorbent typing pad helps reduce fan noise of the quieter laser-type printers.

Dust

If you work at home, you will need to clean your own office machines, one more job you probably wouldn't do at the office. Since designers know that equipment buyers seldom clean their own equipment, style sometimes wins out over functionality. Printers produce and gather dust that must be removed if the machine (and its operator) are to function properly. Note, before buying, whether a printer is covered with tiny grooves that will require a baby's toothbrush to dust.

Speed

Once you've dealt with the truly important ergonomic printer questions introduced above, think about speed.

First-time computer users are often surprised to learn that you don't print only finished work. In fact, you will probably produce more draft versions than ever before simply because it's so easy to do so. If one hundred words per minute was fast on a typewriter, it's crawling on a computer printer where speeds ten times faster are common. Once the thrill of liberation from the typewriter wears off, your printer inevitably begins to seem slow. The question becomes, how long are you willing to wait for each draft? The newer laser printers offer a real solution to the speed bottleneck.

Hewlett Packard
Vancouver Division
P.O. Box 8906
Vancouver, Washington 98668
(800) 354 7622

Portable printer with small footprint

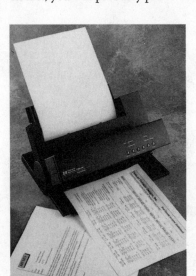

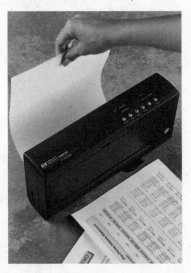

Disks, Fans and Cables

All hard disk drives are fast—the main ergonomic problem is the constant whine produced by the drive itself. You will need to live with that noise all day. Most computer stores are noisy, the worst possible environment for evaluating a hard drive. Try to check it out in a quiet environment, similar to your office.

If you must choose a noisy drive, consider ways to quiet it when you put it to work. Try a sound-absorbent typing pad directly under the computer or external drive. Computer ads aside, there is no reason to keep an external hard disk next to your computer.

Don't hesitate to use an extension cable to move the whine far from your desk. You can usually move the drive up to eighteen feet safely; check the maximum permitted extension with the manufacturer.

Fans

The entire computer system must become quieter. For the moment fans are necessary to cool heat-producing chips, hard disk drives and laser printers. But remember, with each new device, you add additional fan noise to your office. *Listen* carefully to your equipment before you buy it and if it's too loud, look for a quieter alternative.

Cables

Computer manufacturers are beginning to realize that cables can be consolidated. They may even, eventually, be eliminated by using infrared or radio controlled devices which have yet to be perfected. A simple cable plan will save the back of your desk from turning into a jungle of knotted wire. Color coding with plastic tape will differentiate same-color cables. Desks with slots and compartments for hiding cables provide a tidy but pricey ergonomic solution. Be certain you can disconnect a device without disassembling your desk.

Solutions to cable problems

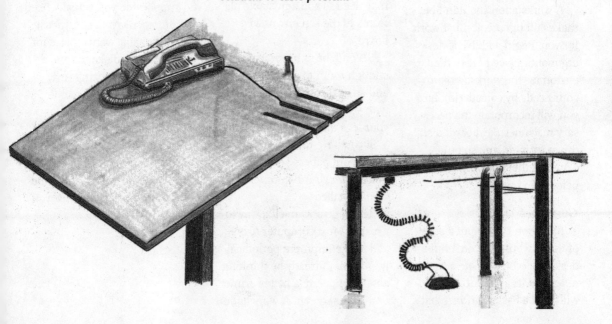

The Computer Workstation

The computer workstation came out of nowhere. Who would have thought twenty years ago that the furniture of science fiction films would suddenly appear in millions of offices. Yet the computer workstation remains one of the most misunderstood accessories in the office. Furniture catalogs routinely pass off flimsy masonite tables with spindly, folding legs and a single narrow shelf as a "complete" workstation. Sure, your PC will work on one, but can you? With no space for your knees or wrists, no way to adjust the distance between your eyes and the screen and no place for files, coffee cups, a mouse or a task light, you can expect to suffer every time you sit down to work.

A workstation shouldn't be makeshift or cute, it must work for you. Begin with basic desk ergonomics (see p. 121), then customize the workstation to your needs by considering how you will incorporate the necessary machines (keyboard, disk drives, printer, and so on). Consider the following caveats before you buy.

Guidelines

First, don't try to put a state-of-the-art computer on a flimsy desk. To accommodate a computer and its accessories, you will need a basic platform that's considerably deeper and sturdier than a normal desk. If your keyboard and computer lack elevation adjustments and won't tilt or swivel, consider a workstation that incorporates these adjustments—the elegant solution. Otherwise, for the sake of your neck and shoulders, you may need to add adjustable platforms to the screen and keyboard.

Second, be sure you have enough room to wiggle around and stretch your legs. Be honest with yourself: can you cross your legs under the tabletop? Will you have plenty of room to spread out papers and personal items *after* your equipment has been installed?

Third, give yourself a way to expand. Most computer users add new equipment periodically. You may already be thinking about a modem, a better printer or a larger screen. A workstation must be able to grow; the more modular and movable everything is, the better.

Fourth, "minor details" like noise and glare can become major problems if you don't deal with them immediately. Avoid white furniture and glossy reflective surfaces. Plan the routing of cables so they don't turn into spaghetti. Remember, just one loose cable can trip a passerby and yank the whole computer onto the floor. Workstations that provide a hidden cable channel in the tabletop are a great blessing. Cable clamps, while less aesthetically pleasing, fasten bundles of cables directly to the edges of a desk, where they will be safe and out of the way.

Fifth, focus on "inner circle" storage. Which computer-related supplies do you actually need within reach? At the very least you'll probably want a place for printer paper, diskettes and a few manuals. Figuring in a mouse pad helps determine how much extra desk space you will need. Each one of these items requires its own shelf, space or drawer. Settle that quickly or you will be surrounded by random clutter while you work.

Workstation Accessories

Floating monitor stand

Cable cutouts or built-in wiring

Vertical storage for manuals

Shelf for printer and paper

Compartments for diskettes

Adjustable keyboard shelf

Mouse pad

Expandable system

Choosing Your Computer Desk

Few things can undermine a project more thoroughly than a wobbly desk. For starters, the basic desk must easily accommodate a large computer system as well as a floating monitor stand, itself capable of supporting two hundred pounds. The monitor stand must glide to any position above the desktop with a flick of the hand. You move a book when you read it, why not your monitor?

You should be able to add or subtract shelves, drawers, equipment stands and adjoining pieces. You will find uniformly matte surfaces restful, particularly if you work in a brightly lighted room. The most ergonomic workstations manage all electrical connections. Power cords, concealed in a generous hidden channel, are held in place with thick rubber grommets. The desk itself plugs into the wall and supplies electricity through surface-mounted outlets. The entire work surface should adjust from twenty-five to thirty inches with levelers on all four legs to compensate for uneven floors.

The Knoll Group
105 Wooster Street
New York, New York 10012
(212) 343 4000

Workstation Errors

Avoid these common mistakes:

Too high. Don't use a fixed desk that is too high for the keyboard.

Computer Desk Ergonomics

Put the keyboard on an adjustable platform or table that is lower than your main desktop.

Find a way to make the monitor adjustable. It should move up and down and be capable of tilting and swiveling until the perfect personal viewing angle is found. If you're sharing equipment, be certain that these adjustments are easy to do.

Locate the printer so that you can easily reach the paper output from your desk.

Put a soft sound-absorbent pad under the printer.

Choose a desk that is wide enough for a pointing device, like a mouse, as well as a copy stand, reference books and papers. You have a right to clutter your own space.

Allow plenty of room on the desktop to move your keyboard. Make sure you have enough desk space *in front of the computer*—not only to comfortably accommodate your forearms and the keyboard but to move both freely. Be sure your keyboard cable is long enough to put the keyboard on your lap while you rest your feet on the desk.

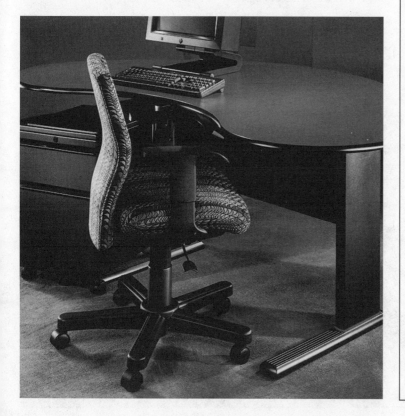

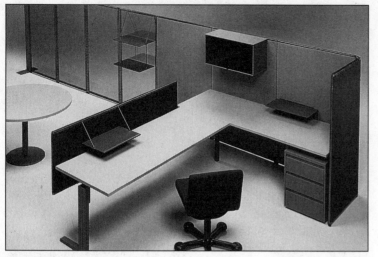

Unifor, Inc.
International Design
Center Two
Suite 706
30-20 Thomson Avenue
Long Island City, NY 11101

Too narrow. Don't use a desk that is too narrow for a mouse plus books and papers.

Too shallow. Avoid shallow "economy workstations" with barely enough room for a tucked-in computer. You're better off with a simple flat table with enough room to move a

keyboard and to spread out your necessary desk clutter. Remember, you have a right to put your feet on the desk.

Too shiny. Do you want to be blinded by your desk?

Difficult to adjust. Be careful of desks that require a manual, tools, more than one person, crawling on the floor, or a degree in mechanical engineer-

ing to make simple adjustments.

Add up the footprints of the computer, modem, monitor, extra disk drives, printer and other peripherals. If the machines are crowding you, first make sure you need them at hand, then consider a larger workstation.

Anthro Technology Furniture
10450 S.W. Manhasset Drive
Tualatin, Oregon 97062
(800) 325 3841

All tools within easy reach

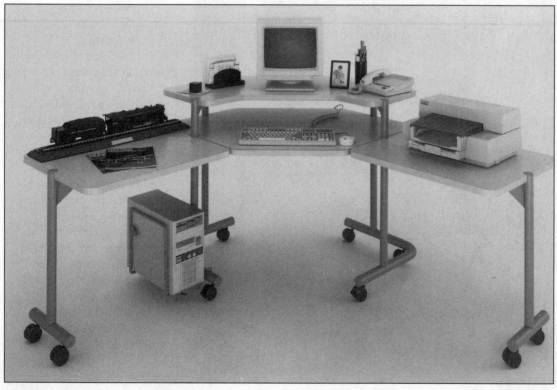

II. The Information-Age Habitat

One of the most important activities that goes on in your habitat is communicating with others. Communications ergonomics deals with purely mechanical questions: easy-to-use push buttons, standard keypad layouts, the comfort and fidelity of earphones, and the accessibility of electronic mail and fax systems. ❦ It also focuses on the process of communication itself, showing how to avoid the devastating "accidents" that come with the new generation of electronic tools. ❦ The stakes are high: will you be enriched or victimized by the communications explosion?

[His] home office . . . contains one thermos of coffee, two laser printers, three personal computers, four telephone/modem lines, and 500 little, yellow sticky Post-its, each screaming with its own reminder. He's often talking on the phone while responding to E-mail and printing out a newsletter—and thinking about something else entirely. The only problem is that deBronkart has trouble getting anything done. The smallest bit of incoming information, the quickest fleeting thought or the slightest peep from a family member has the potential to derail deBronkart from whatever work he should be doing. He might not get back to the task at hand for hours, days, weeks.—EVAN I. SCHWARTZ, "Interrupt-Driven," *Wired*, June 1994, p. 46, San Francisco. Copyright © 1994, Wired Ventures Ltd. All rights reserved.

Information Overload

Cramming speedy new tools into the office without considering how they will affect people produces a peculiar modern affliction: *information overload.* Everywhere you look, piles of mail and messages demand attention.

We are addicted to information, but we deny the ergonomic consequences of our habit. The more information we move, the greater the potential for colossal breakdowns in communication. Even when millions of dollars are at stake, worldwide electronic mail networks can't seem to avoid getting bogged down in petty arguments called "flaring" or "flaming."

Electronic correspondence eats up hours of our time. Deals are lost. Networks flounder in irrelevant details and missed connections. Messages go astray, yet we plunge on in our quest for still more information, denying all the while that any problem exists.

Two familiar traps await: complete communications breakdown and information overload. To avoid them, you must understand these essential ergonomic communication concepts: trust, bandwidth, two-way or one-way communication, media transformation and record keeping.

Building Trust

The Japanese success formula begins with their mastery of communication. Virtually every major undertaking is preceded by a flurry of meetings that puzzle most Westerners, simply because no real decisions ever seem to be made. We in the West emphasize saving time and making quick decisions, while the Japanese work on establishing trust. Whether negotiating or collaborating, we try to eliminate small talk and get right down to business. However, when the time comes for us to sign a contract and actually move forward, we find we are dealing with strangers. We then pass the deal to lawyers, accountants, agents, and advisers, and the offstage sparring begins. Communication between the principals abruptly grinds to a halt; perhaps the whole project is called into question. Without trust, we simply cannot go forward. This is why the Japanese insist on face-to-face meetings before beginning any project. Their single goal, whether people work in different cities or on different shifts, is to establish trust and consensus on important issues. Only then does the astonishingly fast and effective execution of decisions, for which the Japanese are famous, become possible.

Once trust is established, people can separate and begin to draw on an army of electronic tools to work with one another. Whether your co-workers are in other cities or on separate shifts in the same building, it always pays to establish a good working relationship face-to-face before you reach for the fax.

Overload Symptoms

You're harassed by the telephone whenever you sit down to work; phone messages pile up on your desk.

Your mail becomes an avalanche of memos, reports and newsletters; flipping on the computer just makes things worse because your e-mail in-box is always overflowing.

The new fax machine inundates you with junk faxes.

You are constantly interrupted.

You hide at home or in a cafe just to find time to concentrate.

You do your best thinking in airplanes.

The people in your office are avoiding each other's machines.

One-Way or Two-Way?

When trust is solid, the next question becomes, do I need to use an interactive medium? If the answer is yes, the choices are personal meeting or video, audio or computer conferencing. These are listed in diminishing order; the less contact between people, the narrower the communication "bandwidth."

Face-to-face meetings convey subtleties of emotion through a host of nonverbal gestures. Much more than your basic message is communicated. A telephone call reduces the bandwidth to the spoken word. A posted letter shrinks the bandwidth to the written word with no personal contact. Communication by computer network narrows the bandwidth still further—no personal contact or personally written copy.

When to Disappear

How much time do you waste communicating every day? Negotiating, brainstorming, selling, interviewing, solving problems, developing consensus, and getting to know people require two-way communication. Memos, scheduling and ordering usually do not. Avoid the most common mistake: using a two-way medium, such as a personal meeting or the phone, for a simple one-way message. This

---

Communications Media

In descending order of bandwidth:

1. **Two-way**
   face-to-face meetings

2. **Two-way**
   video conference

3. **Two-way**
   audio conference,
   telephone call

4. **Two-way or one-way**
   computer conference

5. **One-way**
   mail, E-mail and fax

---

wasteful habit simply generates meaningless small talk. Use fax or E-mail. If you must call, do so when you can be certain that your contact's answering machine is taking calls.

Should It Go on the Record?

Do you create hidden work for yourself every time you pick up the telephone? In choosing a communications medium, think about whether you want to *record* the exchange. Is a note on a pink telephone slip enough. Does the information need to be shared with others? Is it confidential?

Changing one human communications mode into another in order to create useful information that can be shared and stored is one of the most time-consuming parts of office work. Every step you can eliminate from the process, known as *media transformation,* will save time and money.

Here's how it works: If you begin with oral dictation, the material must be typed and ultimately filed. This takes three steps. Telephone conversations yield notes, which also must be typed and filed. Electronic mail and computer conferencing have a tremendous advantage since they *originate* in a recorded form, which is automatically filed and distributed. The more media transformation steps, the more distorted your information is likely to become.

Think about storage before you drop a communication into the void. Do you need a complete, verbatim record? Are you and your co-workers comfortable typing? Computer conferencing occurs in real time, which permits several participants to be on-line at the same time. You avoid having to set up a face-to-face meeting. Best of all, participants have a complete record of the meeting immediately without any media transformation.

Escaping Telephone Terror

Are you bullied by your telephone? Do you drop everything, interrupt meetings and break into a run whenever the telephone rings?

How much time does it take to get back to work afterward and how many of your telephone calls are truly essential?

Don't subordinate your needs to the demands of a machine. Your telephone calls cannot become the highest priority every moment of the day. A great many telephone calls convey one-way communication which is perfectly suited for an answering machine or fax. Even telephone meetings require time away from the telephone. They work out better if you take a moment to collect your thoughts and look through a few files before you talk.

Rank your telephone calls. Some are urgent; most are not. The main ergonomic issue is control: you should manage the telephone, it should not manage you. Use your answering machine not only to screen calls but to announce when you prefer to *take* telephone calls. Electronic call screening, now available in most parts of the country, permits you to view the telephone number of the caller before answering the telephone.

If, however, you love to talk on the telephone and welcome interruptions—if you actually get a lot done by permitting the telephone to rule your day— there's no reason to change your habits.

Choosing a Telephone

Telephones are still designed for the time when they were new, costs were high and long calls were rare. Using a tool that forces you to hold your arm up to your ear for more than a few minutes is wretched ergonomics. If you spend all day grabbing a telephone and clamping it against your shoulder with the side of your head, your body will pay. Expect a sore neck, aching shoulder and arm, a painful upper back and a red ear. Want to take notes and look up things while you talk? Your body will hurt more.

The alternatives contain compromises with their own ergonomic drawbacks. Try them anyway if you need relief, and don't settle for a difficult machine. The telephone is simply too important for manufacturers to continue ignoring ergonomics.

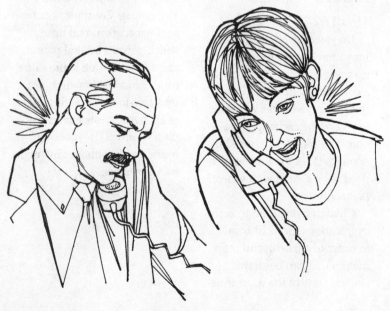

Speakerphones

Although speakerphones make you sound like you're in a train station and often force you to share every conversation with the whole office, they have indisputable ergonomic advantages. You can talk on the telephone without using your hands, thus saving your neck. Also, you can move around, which is always good for your body. Speakerphones work best in a private room.

Cordless Telephones

Ergonomic by its very nature, the cordless telephone permits you to walk around or simply get comfortable while you talk. The high failure rate is due primarily to the same flimsy construction that undermines so many fashionable telephones. Rugged construction is particularly important because a cordless phone inevitably receives rougher treatment than a desk-top model. Look for a rubberized antenna, a far more durable solution than the bare metal variety. A cordless phone must have the same ergonomic features as a regular telephone to be an effective tool.

When the phone's batteries give out abruptly, often midway through a telephone call, you lose your connection. The recharging apparatus must be ergonomic—convenient and easy to use—or else your phone will become little more than an annoying toy. Models in which the entire phone must be returned to the base for recharging have limited mobility and battery life. Double-battery models permit you to recharge a spare battery at the base while you use the phone elsewhere. Switch batteries once a week or so and leave the phone wherever you like at the end of the day.

Cordless telephones use tiny radio transmitters, which determine the range and privacy features. Ten-channel models are more private and effective at extended distances than the

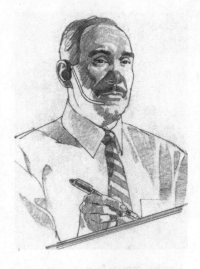

basic two-channel varieties. Very-high-frequency models, operating above 900 megahertz, permit you to extend the range of a cordless far beyond standard telephones.

Consider what it will be like to use your cordless phone while you work. Pocket-size phones or those with belt hooks offer significant ergonomic advantages.

 Sony Electronics Inc.
1 Sony Drive
Park Ridge, New Jersey 07656
(201) 930 1000

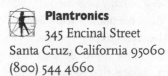 **Plantronics**
345 Encinal Street
Santa Cruz, California 95060
(800) 544 4660

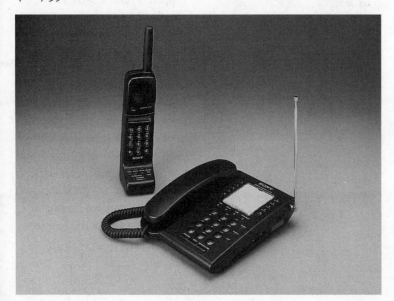

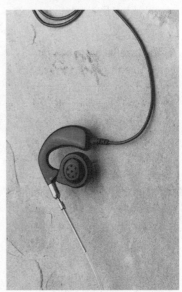

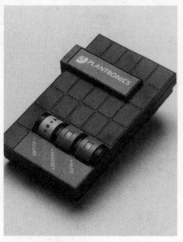

Headset control box

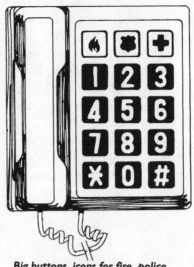

Big buttons, icons for fire, police and ambulance

Headsets

Wearing a headset will maintain your privacy and the audio quality of the call. Yes, you will look like an insect, with an earphone in your ear and wires in your hair, but your hands will be free and your neck and back will thank you. Try a headset if you're hurting. (Forget about borrowing anybody else's headset—it's shaky hygiene.)

Also, telephones with dedicated headset circuits operate much more smoothly than standard models that require manual switching for each call.

Push Buttons

The twelve basic buttons constitute the most essential ergonomic component of the telephone. On the standard push-button telephone, they have an unmistakably satisfying feel. Keys are sculpted to your finger-tips, offering just enough resistance and audio feedback (a slight click) with each button press. Buttons are spaced generously enough so that you don't hit more than one by mistake. Try a basic telephone so you can

---

Telephone Ergonomics

Use your answering machine (or voice-mail system) ruthlessly.

Set phone hours, and let people know about them.

Use a headset or speakerphone if you need your hands for other tasks while on the telephone or if you spend long hours on the phone.

Don't hug the receiver between your cheek and neck. Shoulder stands are nearly useless.

Speed dialing, while useful, works best if the dialed number can be displayed.

Be careful of button mania and shiny, round controls. Your fingers shouldn't slip and slide every time you make a call.

Use a cordless telephone.

Consider oversize buttons and numbers if you are visually impaired, amplified sound if you're hard of hearing.

---

feel the difference before you test more complex solutions. Reject any unit in which the twelve standard buttons become difficult to use.

 AT&T
P.O. Box 3111
Shreveport, Louisiana 71130-9910
(800) 225 3000

New-Age Telephones

For the most part cute, new-age telephones are ergonomic failures. Deregulation, otherwise so welcome, unleashed an avalanche of flimsy gadgetry on the staid old telephone market. Like videocassette recorders, cameras and car radios, the new phones suffer from button mania, the tendency to pack in clusters of useless features that cannot be operated by normal human hands. Flashing lights and microscopic displays compete with mushy rounded buttons that send your fingers careening off sides of the telephone every time you attempt to dial. You fish for each key only to find it difficult to depress properly. Your fingers aren't too big; the keys are too small.

Check a telephone to see if the earpiece actually fits over your ear. Many do not. Test the acoustics on an actual call. Don't be surprised if you have trouble hearing or being heard. Beware of a gap between the time you press a key and hear a tone (delayed tonal feedback). Avoid shiny, glare-producing keys and quirky cradles that don't easily accept the handset.

Electronic Meetings

You've seen fancy satellite interviews on television; should you actually consider something similar for your business? Setting up, even renting, a video conference room is costly, and coordinating the actual conference with participants in two or three places can stretch your resources. You'll need to train a camera operator and rehearse with your staff—people who are "mike shy" will probably be camera shy.

Nonetheless, through video conferencing you can convey a richness of information, complete with shared graphics and a host of nonverbal cues, that rivals a personal meeting. When considering the video conference, think about how expensive travel can be. Train your people to overcome their camera shyness and you may be able to eliminate your next business trip altogether.

Audio (Telephone) Conferencing

Easily arranged multicity audio conferences can be a powerful tool, especially if you attend to the ergonomic requirements before beginning one. First, consider a purely mechanical issue: three voices work best; many more and everyone gets confused. Second, good sound quality, a rare feature in new-age telephones, is essential.

Now for the process of communication. Discipline during meetings must be maintained to avoid confusion; the key issue is the order of speaking. In face-to-face meetings, visual signals usually aid in determining who speaks and who goes next. With three or more people in a telephone conference you may not even know who is speaking, much less who wants to speak next. By making one of the participants a facilitator who will identify each speaker and assure everybody a turn, you can clarify the situation.

The mechanical solution to this problem is voice-activated microphones that permit only one person to speak at a time. Unfortunately, this removes all spontaneity from the conference and causes ugly interruptions when somebody coughs or sneezes. Make sure your conferencing telephones are equipped with mute buttons. Audio conferences work best when the participants know one another well and meet often.

Computer Conferencing

An incredibly powerful communications tool with virtually unlimited possibilities, computer conferencing may make the office itself obsolete. Dozens, even hundreds of people, can share information over any distance. Notes are stored and shared automatically as they are typed, providing one-step media transformation, a powerful tool for people who need to collaborate over great distances. Information stored on the network can be read when convenient. The message you send abroad from Los Angeles at 2:00 PM (10:00 PM London time) will be waiting on-line when the London office opens the next morning. Meet on-line whenever you feel like it, reviewing material from other exchanges while remaining in your office with all your files.

Computer conferencing has two limitations. First, it helps to be a good typist. Second, working with people you can't see or hear, whose handwriting never appears before you and who you never plan to meet in person, is a sure recipe for bizarre communication accidents. Beware of trouble during electronic meetings. Without verbal or visual cues, miscommunication can occur and ordinary ex-changes can escalate quickly into on-line arguments known as "flaming."

Flaming and Groupthink

Don't try to control *flaming* on-line. It's astonishing just how effective the Japanese meeting techniques described on p. 176 can be in resolving what seems like a hopeless situation. Start with a wide communication bandwidth, then narrow it once trust has been established. If possible, meet in person at the beginning of a project. Telephone conversations are the next best solution. Don't panic when intense flaming threatens to sink an important project; pick up the phone—you may even need to schedule a personal meeting.

Not only do arguments flare up unpredictably without audio and video cues, but agreements can be deceptive. Beware of *groupthink*, an Orwellian concept that refers to the way people sometimes arrive at a false sense of consensus.

Temporarily widening the communication bandwidth will generally put things back on track. Again, you may need to meet face-to-face.

On-line, with thousands of details at your fingertips, it's tempting to do nothing at all, a symptom of information overload. Take a deep breath and look again at your choices.

User Interface

During electronic conferencing you will need to think about your chair, keyboard, lighting and other computer-related items. However, the most important ergonomic consideration, the group communications software known as *the user interface* is often ignored in the rush for speed and power. Resist the temptation to buy a feature-laden program that offers "more for your money." An overly complex user interface will plunge your work

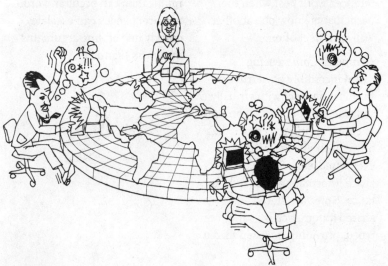

Face-to-Face

Use personal meetings:
At the beginning of a project
When there is distrust
In conflict situations
When the project is poorly defined
When political obstacles appear
When participants represent different cultures, languages or age groups
When dealing with heated emotions

group into chaos day after day, cutting communication to zero (an all too common networking problem when ergonomics is ignored). Remember that each feature comes with a learning curve that *everyone* on your network must master. A confusing user interface means that you must be ready at all times to telephone a befuddled colleague in Sydney, Australia, and walk him through the program. Choose a well-known program that's easy to learn and use.

Before buying, test the user interface on-line: Can records be browsed? How difficult is it to get from one place to another? Can you send documents from your word processor, database and spreadsheet without going though a complicated conversion process? Is it easy to leave (drop) a conference?

Electronic Mail

E-mail may someday replace the postal system once a serious ergonomic problem has been addressed—you must pass though three levels of software to send a message:

1. The original computer software;

2. Modem software;

3. The E-mail system that often bears little similarity to the one on your computer.

Editing and Formatting

On-line editing is clumsy, formatting primitive. So the ergonomic question becomes, How much of your message will actually get through?

To find out, test an E-mail system by sending *yourself* a few letters before you send one to anyone else. Are the margins where you expect them to be? Does the text look right? Are any words or sentences actually missing? E-mail systems on Delphi, Compuserve and Internet are aware of the problem, even if users generally are not, and new systems like America Online with more ergonomic software are in the works.

For now, be certain you have identified and solved every compatibility problem before you commit to an E-mail system.

E-mail Discipline

Select
an intuitive user interface

Beware
of information overload

Check
your formatting

Keep track
of hourly charges

Compose
messages off-line

Invest
in a fast modem

Managing Time On-Line

Electronic mail not only puts you in touch with far-flung individuals but also with a mainframe computer that has enormous storage facilities. Suddenly, all the world's knowledge seems to be just a mouse click away. However, the thrill of accessing vast libraries of data without leaving your office can fade quickly when the phone bill arrives. It's easy to spend hours on-line sifting through mountains of information. Not only does the clock keep running while you retrieve personal messages, but your other work can suffer. Electronic mail requires discipline and a firm hand on the pocketbook.

Fax Machines

The recent fax explosion demonstrates one of the most unfortunate tendencies in consumer electronics: turning a simple device into a hopelessly complex one. Facsimile machines succeeded precisely because their basic operation is ergonomic. In the beginning there were three steps: insert a document, dial the number, then press a large well-marked *send* button. Receiving was completely automatic.

New Features—
Can You Actually Use Them?

Then came the other features, the ones most individuals and small businesses might need once a month or once a year: polling, multiple station send, halftone reproduction, remote terminal identification, and so on. These are implemented via complicated sets of double- and triple-function phone-pad keys.

For example, on one of the most popular brands, you press *send* to send a message, *talk* to talk afterward. However, to print a pass code on the message, you must press *function*, 3, #, #, 1, then *send* and *clear*.

Timers, polling and activity reports are equally daunting. The assumption seems to be that infrequently used features should be more difficult than standard ones. This is entirely

wrong; in fact, you're *less likely* to remember a long command if it's not used often. Should you need to poll remote stations twice a day, you are expected to program a machine, manual in hand, that you initially purchased for its simplicity.

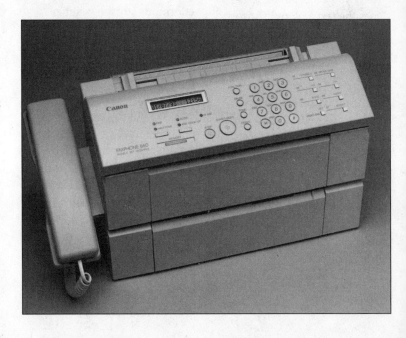

Canon USA
1 Canon Plaza
Lake Success, New York 11042
(516) 328 5149

The Essential Fax

On an unergonomic fax a button labeled *2* is also meant to be used as part of various complex command strings. To do anything beyond simply dialing the number *2*, you must study the manual. With new capabilities appearing regularly, the question becomes, how do you keep a simple machine simple?

The way out of the thicket is not to limit features or cover the machine with tiny buttons but to assign priorities to various tasks. Thus, often-used features like *send* and *talk* can keep their large dedicated buttons while each of the less frequently used features are assigned a single button, say, *polling*, and moved to a hidden subpanel.

Virtually any command can be executed with large, color-coded, labeled buttons that are dedicated to a single function. In a dedicated push-button system a red button labeled *on*

tions does a menu-driven machine make sense.

The Bundled Fax— An Ergonomic Disaster?

In an effort to sell more machines, fax manufacturers

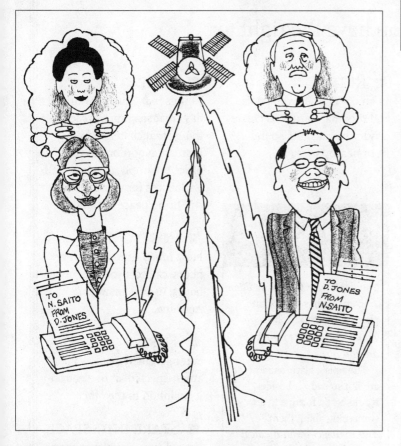

Like E-mail, faxing is a narrow-bandwidth medium that is subject to unfortunate communication accidents.

turns the machine on and off, while infrequently used buttons are concealed beneath a sub-panel. If a machine is simple enough to be operated by dedicated push buttons, it should be. The computer never was. Menu-driven command structures simplify complex machinery, but they complicate simple machines. Only in very large-scale or complex faxing opera-

have developed another bad habit: a tendency to combine in one machine the functions of three or four. Thus, a fax machine can also be a telephone with too many buttons, a second-rate answering machine and a third-rate copier.

Apart from the obvious compromises, it is poor ergonomics to combine machines that are liable to fail at different times. When your third-rate copier jams, you must be prepared to do without a fax or answering machine.

OFFICE WORKER'S
Bill of Rights

You have the right to:

❦ SPRAWL
Put your feet up and work with a keyboard in your lap if you feel like it. Don't allow machines to cramp your style.

❦ MOVE
Sitting in a fixed position for hours brings on everything from headaches to cold feet.

❦ CLUTTER
Are books, papers and desk-top tools part of your job? If it suits your style, you're entitled to surround yourself with disarray.

❦ WRIGGLE
Lie down on the floor and stretch. Take a walking meeting or go for a picnic lunch outside. Work at your stand-up desk for a while. Your body at work needs exercise.

❦ SEE
You'll get far more work done with glare-free ambient light and adjustable task lighting.

❦ RETREAT
In an open office white noise and modular partitions create privacy by masking sound from nearby workers.

Excuses for Continuing to Suffer

You don't want to buck tradition.
Everyone has always complained about this job.
You found a way to work around it.
The noise, glare, shadow, etc. are not so bad . . . besides, it would cost a fortune to do something about them.
You manage—with medical assistance.
My pill/chiropractor/doctor will get me through.
You blame a scapegoat.
The boss doesn't care about my working conditions, so what can I do?
You blame yourself.
It's my own fault for not sitting up straight, getting more sleep, and so on.
You procrastinate.
I'll fix it as soon as I get finished with this project.
You're a masochist.
There's no gain without pain.

❦ HEAR
Things that whine or hum all day create as much anxiety as things that clatter and bang. Insulating portions of your office or simply adding sound enclosures for your machines will bring peace of mind.

❦ POSTPONE
How much time does every phone call cost you? Set phone hours; use an answering machine.

❦ THRIVE
You're entitled to know about any suspected air or electronic pollution in the office.

❦ STARE INTO SPACE
Long-distance focusing every twenty or thirty minutes is essential eye care.

Epilogue: Things That Move

Whether at home or in the office, our minds thrive on variation and our bodies require movement. No tool and no piece of furniture will allow us to remain in the same position for long periods of time without paying a penalty. ❦ We are, after all, animals, and not too long ago our lives required constant movement. Now we have a life of riding and waiting, sitting and watching. We climb on the lawn mower, we sit passively in front of the television and computer. We hold onto labor-saving devices and flick a switch. We remain perfectly still while being entertained. Some part of the mind might be exercised, but the body's muscles, tendons and nerves atrophy. ❦ We are entering a world in which exercise, indeed movement itself, is becoming an option; everywhere we look we are served by machines. But no matter how efficiently things happen, the ergonomic challenge will remain the same: to satisfy the most essential needs of the body. The more sedentary life becomes, the more we will need ergonomic solutions that permit us to move. Even a bed must allow a range of movement to provide restful sleep. ❦ Bad ergonomics leaves us locked in place by an indifferent machine, passive and stiff, depressed and aching. Good ergonomics speaks directly to the body. Ten seconds after we begin using an ergonomic tool, we feel the difference. ❦ The rocking chair, which has been with us for hundreds of years, owes its popularity to its soothing movement, which is perfect for nursing a baby or simply relaxing and thinking deeply. It's one of the great, proven ergonomic tools. 🍂 Adjustable reading chairs allow for smooth periodic postural adjustments—the opportunity for *movement* makes all the difference. A new generation of couches transform themselves into recliners. One moment we might be sitting upright and conversing, the next we can be reclining listening to music. All of the movement is smooth and effortless. 🍂 A self-articulating office chair liberates the body from the traditional static working position, leaving us free to scoot around, rock back and forth or stretch vigorously while seated. A cordless phone permits us to walk around while we talk. A walking meeting gets us out of the office altogether, benefiting our eyes while the body is exercised. The ergonomic choice feels better immediately because it permits us to change position at will. 🍂 We all want a relaxed and

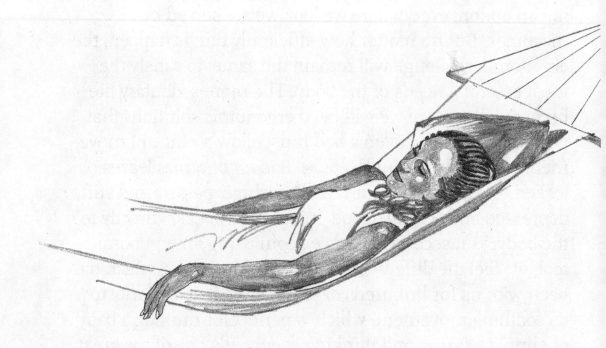

healthy body. That's why the word *ergonomics* has begun to appear so frequently in articles and advertising for everything from computers to furniture, from kitchen and office equipment to automobiles. We simply cannot get along without it anymore. The next generation of ergonomic products will help us move naturally through the mechanized world we have created in our office and home and the real one that lies just outside. ❦ Change, movement and grace. This is a friendly world; we built it, and now we have the tools to live in it on our own terms. We can choose to inhabit healthful, comfortable environments, amicable places that serve our needs. We can be the masters of our own possessions, the actors on a human-centered stage. ❦ We can feel good all day.

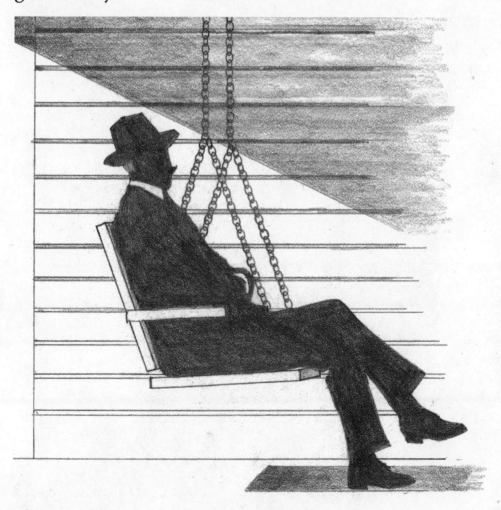

The Authors

Gordon Inkeles's health books, including the classic *The Art of Sensual Massage*, have become standard works throughout the world. He has produced several documentary films and has lectured widely on health and stress control. *Ergonomic Living* continues to emphasize his specialty: the easy-to-learn stress reduction program that readers can take home and use immediately. Inkeles is a charter member of The National Writers Union.

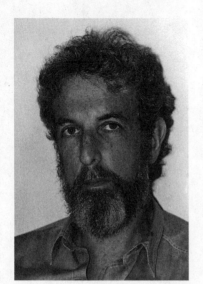

In her career as office automation consultant at SRI International, Iris Schencke began her study of ergonomic trends in Europe and America. She went on to international management at Infomedia, a computer conferencing pioneer. Later, as international product manager at Apple Computer, she worked with a team that introduced ergonomic keyboard design for personal computers. Ms. Schencke has an M.A. from Stockholm University and an M.B.A. from Stanford University.

Both authors live in Arcata, California.

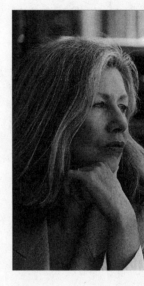